The
Medical
Staff's Guide
to Overcoming
Competence Assessment
Challenges

Carol S. Cairns, CPMSM, CPCS

Sally Pelletier, CPMSM, CPCS

Frances Ponsioen, CPMSM, CPCS

Anne Roberts, CPCS, CPMSM

⊣CPro

The Medical Staff's Guide to Overcoming Competence Assessment Challenges is published by HCPro, Inc.

Copyright © 2013 HCPro, Inc.

All rights reserved. Printed in the United States of America.   5 4 3 2 1

ISBN: 978-1-60146-966-3

HCPro, Inc., provides information resources for the healthcare industry.

HCPro, Inc., is not affiliated in any way with The Joint Commission, which owns the JCAHO and Joint Commission trademarks.

Carol S. Cairns, CPMSM, CPCS, Author

Sally Pelletier, CPMSM, CPCS, Author

Frances Ponsioen, CPMSM, CPCS, Author

Anne Roberts, CPCS, CPMSM, Author

Elizabeth Jones, Editor

Mike Mirabello, Graphic Artist

Matt Sharpe, Senior Manager of Production

Shane Katz, Art Director

Jean St. Pierre, Vice President, Operations and Customer Relations

Advice given is general. Readers should consult professional counsel for specific legal, ethical, or clinical questions.

Arrangements can be made for quantity discounts. For more information, contact:

HCPro, Inc.

75 Sylvan Street, Suite A-101

Danvers, MA 01923

Telephone: 800-650-6787 or 781-639-1872

Fax: 800-639-8511

Email: *customerservice@hcpro.com*

Visit HCPro online at: *www.hcpro.com* and *www.hcmarketplace.com*

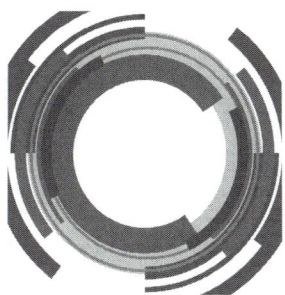

Contents

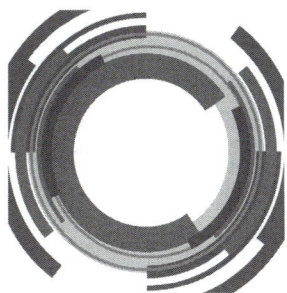

About the Authors

Anne Roberts, CPCS, CPMSM

Anne Roberts, CPCS, CPMSM, is the senior director of medical affairs at Children's Medical Center of Dallas, where she oversees eight departments, with her primary focus being on medical staff services and medical staff quality. Additionally, she is a consultant and speaker with The Greeley Company, a division of HCPro, Inc., in Danvers, Mass. As a recognized expert in the field, she presents frequently for the National Association Medical Staff Services (NAMSS) and other healthcare entities on topics ranging from medical staff credentialing to legal strategies for medical services professionals and medical staff leaders and has numerous guidebooks published by HCPro.

Carol S. Cairns, CPMSM, CPCS

Carol S. Cairns, CPMSM, CPCS, has participated in the development of the medical staff services profession for more than 35 years. She is a senior consultant and frequent presenter with The Greeley Company. A recognized expert in the field, Cairns has been a faculty member with NAMSS since 1990. She presents frequently for NAMSS and other healthcare entities at numerous state and national seminars on subjects such as basic and advanced credentialing and privileging, core privileging, AHP credentialing, the Centers for Medicare & Medicaid Services' *Conditions of Participation*, and the standards of—and survey preparation for—The Joint Commission, the National Committee for Quality Assurance, and the Healthcare Facilities Accreditation Program.

Sally Pelletier, CPMSM, CPCS

Sally Pelletier, CPMSM, CPCS, is an advisory consultant and the chief credentialing officer for The Greeley Company. She brings more than 20 years of credentialing and privileging experience to her work with medical staff leaders and medical services professionals (MSP) across the nation.

Pelletier advises clients in the areas of accreditation, regulatory compliance, credentialing and privileging process simplification and redesign, and medical staff services department operations; she also provides leadership and development training for medical staff leaders and MSPs.

Pelletier began her career in 1992 as the medical staff coordinator at The Memorial Hospital in North Conway, N.H. She has served as secretary and as the Northeast region representative on the board of directors for NAMSS. Other leadership roles for NAMSS have included serving as a NAMSS instructor; and chairing the Governance, Management, and Manpower Committee, the Bylaws Committee, and the Credentialing Elements Task Force. In addition, she served as president of the New Hampshire Association Medical Staff Services, from which she received the 2008 Excellence in Medical Staff Services Award.

Pelletier serves as an expert witness and presents at state and national seminars on a variety of topics related to medical staff leadership training, leading practices in credentialing and privileging, and physician competency management.

She has coauthored several HCPro/Greeley books, including:

- *Core Privileges for Physicians: A Practical Approach to Developing and Implementing Criteria-Based Privileges,* Fifth Edition (2010)

- *Assessing the Competency of Low-Volume Practitioners: Tools and Strategies for OPPE & FPPE Compliance,* Second Edition (2009)

- *The FPPE Toolbox: Field-Tested Documents for Credentialing, Competency, and Compliance* (2008)

- *Core Privileges for AHPs: Develop and Implement Criteria-Based Privileging for Non-Physician Practitioners,* Second Edition (2011)

- *Converting to Core Privileging: 10 Essential Steps to a Criteria-Based Program* (2007)

Frances M. Ponsioen, CPMSM, CPCS

Frances M. Ponsioen, CPMSM, CPCS, is Credence site director for The Greeley Company. She has more than 20 years of experience in medical staff services, most recently serving 10 years as the director of medical staff services for the Baptist Health System in San Antonio, Texas, a five-hospital system. In her roles, she worked directly with medical staff leaders and hospital executives to ensure continued compliance with all regulatory standards related to the medical staff and credentialing responsibilities; she implemented a credentialing software system while transitioning the primary source verification process in-house for the healthcare system; she developed and implemented core privilege forms for medical staff and allied health staff; and she fully reorganized all medical staff governance documents. She also developed a successful plan for the full upgrade and implementation of the credentialing software system, bringing the initial application and reappointment process online and fully electronic.

Ponsioen has served on her local South Texas Association of Medical Staff Professionals as president elect, president, past president, and secretary. She has been a member of NAMSS since 2003 and has served on the Governance Management and Manpower Committee, Nominating Committee, and Audit and Finance Committee, also serving as a director at large. She has been a member of the Texas Association of Medical Staff Services since 1995. In 2007, she received the Joan Covell-Carpenter Award from NAMSS for an article she wrote in the publication *Synergy*.

1

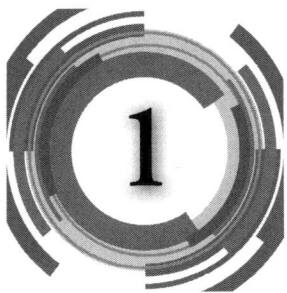

Competence Assessment for Initial Appointment

Anne Roberts, CPCS, CPMSM

CASE STUDY

Dr. Jones has just relocated to the area and joined a large plastic surgery group. He has submitted his application for membership and clinical privileges at the hospital and has requested that the process be expedited so he can provide coverage for his new partners, one of whom will soon be retiring. The practice manager has contacted the CEO of the hospital to ask for assistance in getting Dr. Jones' application pushed through as quickly as possible. As the plastic surgery group produces a lot of revenue for the hospital, the CEO contacts the medical staff services department and reiterates that the application needs to be expedited. These political motivations to expedite an application can often pressure medical services professionals (MSP) to rush through the credentialing and privileging process and push paper rather than performing a thorough quality review of the applicant's education, qualifications, current clinical competence, and prior practice history.

Establishing Minimum Threshold Criteria

During the initial credentialing process, organizations must verify a practitioner's education, licensure, prior practice history (to identify if there have been prior competence concerns), and current clinical competence. The medical staff bylaws and associated policies should clearly delineate the minimum threshold criteria for applicants who apply to provide services at an organization. For practitioners, the minimum threshold credentialing criteria typically includes:

- Graduation from an accredited medical/dental/osteopathic school

- Successful completion of an accredited residency program and additional training in a subspecialty program (if applicable)

- A current, unrestricted state medical/dental/osteopathic license

- A comprehensive criminal background check free of red flags

- Professional liability insurance coverage with minimum limits as required by the organization's governing board

- Documentation of current clinical competence (as described throughout this chapter)

Once a practitioner submits an application, MSPs, who work in the medical staff services department, then verify directly through the primary source (e.g., the medical/dental/osteopathic school, the state licensing board, etc.) all minimum threshold criteria for education and any other credentialing requirements established by the organization. Other criteria for credentialing may include but are not limited to verification of:

- All education, training, and academic appointments

- Status at all prior and/or current hospital or other clinical affiliations

- All prior and/or current employers

- All prior licenses

- Current state and/or federal narcotics registration

- Current peer references

- Claims history

- Review of reports to the National Practitioner Data Bank (NPDB)

- Review of sanctions from the Office of Inspector General

In addition to the minimum threshold criteria for credentialing, organizations must also develop a comprehensive privileging system and establish minimum threshold criteria that a practitioner must meet to prove current clinical competence for each privilege he or she requests. The decision to grant privileges must be an objective, evidence-based process, and the hospital (based on recommendations from the organized medical staff and approval by the governing body) must establish criteria that determine a practitioner's ability to provide patient care, treatment, and services within the scope of the privilege(s) that he or she requests.

The Medical Staff's Guide to Overcoming Competence Assessment Challenges

The first step in developing minimum threshold criteria for clinical privileges is to first identify what privileges the organization will offer in each of the specialty or subspecialty areas. Prior to granting privileges to any practitioner, the organization must determine that the resources necessary to support the requested privileges are currently available or will be available within a specified time frame. Essential information, such as financial resources, equipment, space, and types of personnel necessary to support the requested privilege, must be evaluated as part of the process for establishing minimum threshold criteria.

Once the privileges are established, each department chair recommends to the credentials committee the minimum threshold criteria (i.e., level of education, training, experience, etc.) that are required for applicants to demonstrate that they have the current skills and clinical competence to exercise the requested privileges.

In addition to the minimum threshold criteria, the appropriate department chair must determine the core set of clinical activities that any practitioner with the minimum training required by the organization should be competent to perform. If the organization requires residency training and board certification in the applicable specialty area, the department chair should also evaluate what other criteria the applicant must submit to determine that he or she has the experience needed to demonstrate competence. Some examples include:

- Completion of subspecialty fellowship training (e.g., cardiac anesthesia fellowship, hand surgery fellowship, etc.)

- Documentation of successfully performing X number of specialty-specific procedures in the past X months (e.g., documentation of at least 25 cardiovascular procedures successfully performed within the past 12 months in which the applicant functioned as the primary surgeon)

- Documentation of appropriately treating X number of a specified type of patient in the past X months (e.g., documentation of appropriately treating at least 25 pediatric oncology patients in an inpatient setting within the past 24 months)

Many organizations have also revised their initial case log requirements for applicants who have completed an Accreditation Council for Graduate Medical Education or American Osteopathic Association–accredited training program in the past few years, as the applicant will likely have significant recent clinical experience, which his or her training program director can attest to.

In the case study described at the beginning of this chapter regarding Dr. Jones, the plastic surgeon requesting that his application for membership and clinical privileges be expedited, the organization likely already has the threshold criteria established, and the medical staff services department just needs to review his request to ensure he meets the minimum threshold criteria. If so, the medical staff services department would then begin gathering and verifying the data to confirm current clinical competence. If the applicant, in this case Dr. Jones, does not meet the minimum threshold criteria, the medical staff services department should notify him that he is ineligible for the requested privileges and that his application for membership and request for clinical privileges cannot be processed. Keep in mind that this is not the same thing as denying privileges, which would afford Dr. Jones due process.

Other practitioners to whom your organization grants clinical privileges or permission to provide services (such as allied health professionals or advanced practice professionals) should be treated in the same manner. The organization should outline minimum threshold criteria for each privilege, and the individual should be responsible for providing documentation that proves that he or she is qualified and competent to provide the services requested.

Evaluating Competence

Organizations must evaluate an applicant's ability to perform the privileges that he or she has requested. Competence criteria required by most organizations include but are not limited to the following:

- Appropriate education/training specific to the privileges requested

- Clinical peer references

- Clinical evaluations from prior department chairs and/or training program directors (see section below on developing comprehensive evaluation forms)

- Relevant and recent utilization history (e.g., activity such as admissions, consults, etc.) and quality review results (i.e., has the applicant performed the procedure recently, and what were the clinical outcomes?)

- Case logs from the past 12 to 24 months

- Ongoing professional practice evaluation (OPPE) data

- Board certification in the specialty/subspecialty in which privileges are requested

- Continuing medical education relevant to the privileges requested

- Current health status (Documentation may include the applicant's statement that no health problems exist that could affect his or her practice or an attestation from peers. If there are any current or prior health concerns that could potentially affect the practitioner's ability to perform the requested privileges, then his or her current health status should be evaluated by his or her treating provider to confirm that he or she can competently exercise their existing clinical privileges.)

Burden on the applicant

Once the minimum threshold criteria are set, all individuals requesting that privilege have to provide documentation proving that they meet the eligibility criteria. The burden lies solely on the applicant; it is his or her responsibility to prove that he or she has the current clinical competence required to perform the privileges requested. If an applicant does not meet the minimum threshold criteria, he or she is simply not eligible to apply for the privileges, and his or her application cannot be processed. Or, if the applicant fails to provide requested or sufficient documentation, then the medical staff can deem the application incomplete. Not being eligible to request the privileges or deeming an application incomplete is not a denial of privileges; denying a physician's privileges is reportable to the NPDB and state medical boards, and the practitioner may be entitled to due process if afforded in your bylaws.

Alternatives to deeming an application incomplete

If an organization requires specific case log documentation and an applicant does not meet the requirement, one option, other than deeming the individual ineligible, is to grant the privileges and require precepting. In the case of Dr. Jones, the plastic surgeon in the case study at the beginning of this chapter, if he meets all minimum threshold criteria set by the department for the privileges he has requested with the exception of providing the specified number of cases performed, the organization should determine whether he meets the criteria for precepting. For example, if the criteria for plastic surgery include a requirement to submit documentation of at least 75 plastic surgery procedures relevant to the privileges requested within the past 12 months, and Dr. Jones is able to submit documentation of only 60 cases, the organization may elect to offer precepting for the additional cases.

In general, precepting is a process that allows individuals to "train up" or receive additional training at your organization to obtain the skills and competence necessary to perform specific procedures.

To offer precepting, an organization should have a preceptor policy in place, and the privilege delineation must clearly outline that this is an option (see Chapter 7 for more information on the precepting process and policy requirements). If the medical staff is going to offer precepting, the department chair should add this option as part of its delineation that details the minimum threshold criteria. The following is some example language:

> *"Applicant must provide documentation of performing 75 (X type) procedures in the past 12 months; if the applicant is unable to demonstrate the performance of 75 cases in the past 12 months, the department chair will assign an additional level of focused professional practice evaluation (FPPE) as deemed necessary to demonstrate competence and as outlined in the medical staff policies and procedures. The FPPE may include direct observation, retrospective chart review, or precepting of a specified number of cases."*

See "Competence Assessment Through FPPE After Granting Clinical Privileges" for the steps the department chair should take after the applicant has completed the initial FPPE.

Cross Privileges and Turf Wars

At times, determining the minimum competence criteria can be challenging for medical staff leaders, particularly when a privilege crosses multiple disciplines. For example, vascular rings is a procedure that can be performed by both general surgeons and cardiovascular surgeons. The organization needs to determine whether it will allow both types of surgeons to perform this procedure, and, if so, competence criteria for this procedure should be the same regardless of whether it is performed by a general surgeon or a cardiovascular surgeon.

Most larger organizations have restricted Cesarean section privileges to OB/GYN practitioners; however, some smaller organizations still allow family practitioners who practice obstetrics to request or maintain Cesarean section privileges. If these privileges are extended to both OB/GYNs and family practitioners, equivalent competence criteria for this privilege must be established.

Turf wars or cross-privileging disputes among specialists can often arise and make setting threshold criteria a difficult and cumbersome process. For example, as mentioned above, vascular rings can be performed by general surgeons or cardiovascular surgeons; some organizations have determined that this privilege should be restricted to only cardiovascular surgeons. This can cause a turf war if the general surgeons are not in agreement and feel that they should be allowed to maintain these privileges.

Or, in the other example above, many organizations have had to deal with a turf war related to no longer allowing family practitioners to perform Cesarean sections. Again, this can cause a turf war if the family practitioners feel that they should be allowed to maintain these privileges.

The best way to remedy concerns related to establishing minimum threshold criteria for cross privileges or to address possible turf wars is to ensure that the organization includes all of the individuals who are considered stakeholders in the discussions. When establishing criteria for cross privileges, all departments that will be performing the procedure need to agree on the minimum threshold criteria for competence, because the criteria must be equivalent across all departments performing the procedure. If there is a disagreement on the minimum threshold criteria requirements, the issue and recommendations from all parties should be submitted to the credentials committee and/or medical executive committee (MEC) for review and resolution.

For turf wars that cannot be resolved at the department level, such as between family practitioners and OB/GYNs, the argument/concerns and supporting documentation from all parties should be submitted to the credentials committee or MEC for review and resolution.

For both cross privileges and turf wars, the committee(s) should review the proposals in detail to determine what is considered sufficient evidence of education, training, and experience to demonstrate competence to perform the procedure(s) in question. The committees should take into consideration the recommendations and opinions of all parties and seek further clarification if needed to make an informed decision.

If the request is for a new privilege, then once the committees and the board approve the new criteria for the privilege, applicants can submit a request for said privilege and submit the required competence documentation. If the request is to change the minimum threshold criteria for an already established privilege, then the medical staff will need to review how this change will affect current staff. For example, if the competence criteria become more stringent, the organization will need to review all practitioners who currently hold the privilege to determine whether they will be able to meet the new criteria. If they are unable to meet the criteria, then they no longer qualify for the privilege and should be notified. This is not a reportable action because it is not a restriction of privileges; the practitioners merely no longer meet the established criteria.

In the examples above related to limiting procedures to specific types of practitioners, if the committees and the board approve these limitations, they should notify the practitioners who will be affected that they are no longer eligible for these privileges because the criteria have now changed. A practitioner who currently holds the privilege does not need to withdraw the privilege, as it is not optional; they simply receive notification from the organization of their ineligibility. Again, this is not reportable to the NPDB or state licensing board, as the practitioners merely no longer meet the minimum threshold criteria.

As noted above, these concerns can be very political and have a significant effect on an individual's practice; therefore, it is extremely important to ensure clear communication during the review process to all affected parties and to ensure that all parties have a seat at the table during the discussions. In these instances, the medical staff leaders' recommendation must be focused on what will best serve the patients. Additionally, the committees need to take into consideration when the changes will take effect, as practitioners may already have cases scheduled. The organization needs to ensure that appropriate coverage for those patients is provided by practitioners who meet the new criteria.

Determining Initial Competence for Low- and No-Volume Practitioners

Organizations should proactively identify how they will address low- or no-volume practitioners, both at initial appointment and reappointment, to ensure that they are extending privileges only to individuals who can demonstrate current clinical competence. See Chapter 11 for information on addressing competence challenges related to low- or no-volume practitioners at the time of reappointment.

If an applicant has little to no recent clinical activity and is therefore unable to demonstrate current clinical competence, the organization must determine what options best fit the applicant. Some options for low- and no-volume practitioners at the time of initial appointment include:

- Discuss the practitioner's intent to utilize the privileges requested. Perhaps a different category of privileges, such as refer-and-follow or consult-and-assist privileges, would better fit the applicant's practice. These privilege categories allow the practitioner options to interact with the care team but not serve as the primary care practitioner during a patient's hospital stay. Or, if the applicant anticipates participating only in membership activities, then he or she may not need clinical privileges and may be interested in applying only for staff membership.

- If a practitioner has been out of practice for a significant amount of time or in a private or office-based practice for many years and has no current inpatient experience, the organization may want to consider requiring the practitioner to participate in a refresher course or remedial course. The Federation of State Medical Boards keeps an up-to-date list of these types of courses that are offered across the country, many of which customize training based on need. Many times, if the organization is willing to invest in the practitioner (for example, if a hospital has hired him or her as a hospitalist), it will pay for the course(s). Otherwise, the cost may fall to the practitioner.

- As mentioned earlier, the organization could also elect to require precepting to afford the practitioner the option to receive additional training before granting him or her privileges to provide patient care independently.

Clinical Evaluations

In the past, the only clinical evaluations that some organizations obtained as part of the credentialing process were reference letters from the applicant's peers. This was often looked at as the "buddy system," (as most people are not going to list a peer reference who is going to provide negative feedback), and therefore most organizations have determined that a more meaningful approach is necessary to evaluate an applicant's competence.

One common practice is to get a clinical evaluation from the applicant's residency or fellowship program director if he or she has recently (e.g., within the past five years) completed postgraduate training. During residency or fellowship training, the program director, along with other faculty members who provide supervision during the training program, complete routine evaluations of all residents and fellows. The program director can attest to not only the type of experience the applicant gained during training but also his or her clinical performance during training. If the applicant has recently completed training, the program director can also attest to whether the applicant is qualified and competent to perform the privilege(s) he or she has requested.

In addition to program director evaluations, it is also common practice to obtain a clinical evaluation from the department chair from the applicant's current or most recent primary admitting facility. The department chair can attest to the applicant's performance at the organization and can disclose whether there were any concerns related to the applicant's competence, behavior, or other performance issues.

If the applicant has held a faculty appointment at a university, the medical staff services department can also seek a clinical evaluation from the applicable department chair from the university. A university department chair typically is responsible for overseeing the faculty's overall performance, including not only clinical competence, but also performance as employees, educators, and/or researchers.

CHAPTER 1

Peer reference letters and clinical evaluations must be comprehensive and ask the right questions to cover all pertinent information. Clinical evaluations should include not only questions that solicit information related to utilization or recent clinical experience, but also whether the evaluator is aware of any possible health concerns, behavioral issues, or any other performance concerns. The organization may opt to also include as part of its clinical evaluations an assessment of the six general competencies developed by the Accreditation Council for Graduate Medical Education and the American Board of Medical Specialties and adopted by The Joint Commission:

- Patient care: Practitioners are expected to provide patient care that is compassionate, appropriate, and effective for the promotion of health, prevention of illness, treatment of disease, and care at the end of life.

- Medical/clinical knowledge: Practitioners are expected to demonstrate knowledge of established and evolving biomedical, clinical, and social sciences and the application of their knowledge to patient care and the education of others.

- Practice-based learning and improvement: Practitioners are expected to be able to use scientific evidence and methods to investigate, evaluate, and improve patient care practices.

- Interpersonal and communication skills: Practitioners are expected to demonstrate interpersonal and communication skills that enable them to establish and maintain professional relationships with patients, families, and other members of healthcare teams.

- Professionalism: Practitioners are expected to demonstrate behaviors that reflect a commitment to continuous professional development, ethical practice, an understanding of and sensitivity to diversity, and a responsible attitude toward their patients, their profession, and society.

- Systems-based practice: Practitioners are expected to demonstrate both an understanding of the contexts and systems in which healthcare is provided and the ability to apply this knowledge to improve and optimize healthcare.

If your organization elects to incorporate the six general competencies into its evaluation forms, MSPs should work with their medical staff leaders to draft several questions that fall under each general area. Please see Figure 1.1 for a sample form using the six general competencies.

10   © 2013 HCPro, Inc.   **The Medical Staff's Guide to Overcoming Competence Assessment Challenges**

FIGURE 1.1
PROFESSIONAL REFERENCE QUESTIONNAIRE

This sample questionnaire may be adapted for a variety of professional references, such as residency/fellowship director, previous healthcare affiliations (e.g., clinical service/department chair), peer recommendations, etc.

[Bracketed information is intended to be instructional to users and therefore should be removed from the form before use.]

Section I

[To be completed by organization requesting the reference]

Name of reference: _____

Professional evaluation concerning: [Applicant's full name, including any other name(s) used]

_____

_____

_____

Specialty/subspecialty:

_____

_____

_____

**Attach
or scan
applicant's
picture here**

We have received an application from the above-named and pictured individual stating that he/she: (indicate as applicable)

❑ completed a residency, internship, fellowship (requesting entity: circle as applicable) at your institution from

___ ___ / ___ ___ to ___ ___ / ___ ___ (MM / YY– MM / YY)

❑ was a staff member at your institution from

___ ___ / ___ ___ to ___ ___ / ___ ___ (MM / YY–MM / YY)

❑ has named you as a professional reference.

FIGURE 1.1

PROFESSIONAL REFERENCE QUESTIONNAIRE (CONT.)

The reference should check the accuracy of the information above, and change or complete as appropriate.

Section II

[To be completed by the individual providing the reference]

Present professional position: _____

My responses are based on (check all appropriate responses)

❏ direct observation.

❏ review of accumulated information and reports about the practitioner's performance.

I know the applicant (check the most accurate response)

❏ very well.   ❏ well.   ❏ casually.   ❏ personally.   ❏ professionally.

❏ I do not personally know the applicant. (If checked, please skip the remaining questions in this section (Reference's relationship with the applicant) and go directly to Section III (Professional knowledge, skills, and attitude.)

Please answer the following questions based on your personal knowledge and direct observations. Your candor is greatly appreciated.

REFERENCE'S RELATIONSHIP WITH THE APPLICANT

1. **How long have you known the applicant?** _____

2. **During what time period did you have the opportunity to directly observe the applicant's practice of medicine?** _____

3. **In what setting(s) did you observe the applicant (e.g., office, hospital, residency program, etc.)?**

    _____

    _____

4. **Was the applicant active in your organization?**

    ❏ Yes   ❏ No

    How frequently did you observe the applicant?

    ❏ Daily   ❏ Weekly   ❏ Monthly   ❏ Infrequently

    Comment:

    _____

    _____

         The Medical Staff's Guide to Overcoming Competence Assessment Challenges

FIGURE 1.1
PROFESSIONAL REFERENCE QUESTIONNAIRE (CONT.)

5. **Was your observation done in connection with any official professional title or position?**

   ❏ Yes   ❏ No

   If so, please indicate title and organization:

   _____

   What was the applicant's title or position?

   _____

6. **Were you previously, are you now, or are you about to become related to the applicant as family or through a professional partnership or financial association?**

   ❏ Yes   ❏ No

   If yes, please explain:

   _____

   _____

   _____

   _____

Section III

PROFESSIONAL KNOWLEDGE, SKILLS, AND ATTITUDE

If you do not have adequate knowledge to answer a particular question, please indicate Unable to evaluate (UE)

1. **For each aspect of performance below, please place an X at the place on the scale between poor and excellent that best describes this provider's typical level of performance:**

Medical knowledge	Excellent	Poor	UE
– Basic medical/clinical knowledge			⊢—⊣
– Knowledge in specialty	⊢—┼—┼—┼—⊣		⊢—⊣
– Technical and clinical skills	⊢—┼—┼—┼—⊣		⊢—⊣

Clinical judgment	Excellent	Poor	UE
– Basic clinical judgment	⊢—┼—┼—┼—⊣		⊢—⊣
– Availability and thoroughness of patient care	⊢—┼—┼—┼—⊣		⊢—⊣
– Appropriate and timely use of consultants	⊢—┼—┼—┼—⊣		⊢—⊣

FIGURE 1.1

PROFESSIONAL REFERENCE QUESTIONNAIRE (CONT.)

	Excellent	Poor	UE
– Quality/appropriateness of patient care outcomes	├──┼──┼──┼──┤		├──┤
– Appropriateness of resource use (e.g., admissions, procedures, length of stay, tests, etc.)	├──┼──┼──┼──┤		├──┤
– Thoroughness of medical record documentation	├──┼──┼──┼──┤		├──┤

Communication skills

– Overall communication skills	├──┼──┼──┼──┤		├──┤
– Verbal and written fluency in English	├──┼──┼──┼──┤		├──┤
– Legibility of medical records	├──┼──┼──┼──┤		├──┤
– Responsiveness to patient needs	├──┼──┼──┼──┤		├──┤

Interpersonal skills

– Ability to work with members of healthcare team	├──┼──┼──┼──┤		├──┤
– Rapport with patients	├──┼──┼──┼──┤		├──┤
– Rapport with families	├──┼──┼──┼──┤		├──┤
– Rapport with hospital staff	├──┼──┼──┼──┤		├──┤

Professionalism

– Timely documentation of medical record	├──┼──┼──┼──┤		├──┤
– Participation in medical staff organization activities (e.g., committees, leadership positions, etc.)	├──┼──┼──┼──┤		├──┤
– Participation in continuing medical education	├──┼──┼──┼──┤		├──┤
– Demonstration of ethical standards in treatment	├──┼──┼──┼──┤		├──┤
– Maintenance of patient confidentiality	├──┼──┼──┼──┤		├──┤
– Fulfillment of emergency department call responsibilities	├──┼──┼──┼──┤		├──┤

The Medical Staff's Guide to Overcoming Competence Assessment Challenges

FIGURE 1.1
PROFESSIONAL REFERENCE QUESTIONNAIRE (CONT.)

2. Upon review of the applicant's request for clinical privileges and criteria, as applicable, (enclosed), do you find the privileges requested to be appropriate and in keeping with your knowledge of the applicant's experience and clinical activity at your organization?

❑ Yes ❑ No

If no, please explain:

_____

_____

_____

3. Have you ever observed or been informed of any physical, mental, emotional, or behavioral issues the applicant has or had that could potentially affect his/her ability to exercise all or any of the privileges requested or to perform the duties of medical staff appointment?

❑ Yes ❑ No ❑ No information

If yes, please explain:

_____

_____

_____

4. To the best of your knowledge, have any of the following ever been denied, challenged, investigated, terminated, reduced, not renewed, limited, withdrawn from or resignation submitted, suspended, revoked, modified, placed on probation, relinquished, or voluntarily surrendered, or do you have knowledge of any such actions that are pending?

• License or registration	❑ Yes	❑ No	❑ No information
• Clinical privileges	❑ Yes	❑ No	❑ No information
• Hospital appointment	❑ Yes	❑ No	❑ No information
• Affiliation with any healthcare organization	❑ Yes	❑ No	❑ No information
• Professional status	❑ Yes	❑ No	❑ No information
• Employment arrangement with any healthcare facility	❑ Yes	❑ No	❑ No information
• Employment arrangement with a physician group	❑ Yes	❑ No	❑ No information

---

FIGURE 1.1

PROFESSIONAL REFERENCE QUESTIONNAIRE (CONT.)

    If yes, please explain:

    _____

    _____

    _____

5.   **Do you know of any malpractice action instituted or in process against the applicant?**

    ❏ Yes   ❏ No   ❏ No information

    If yes, please explain:

    _____

    _____

    _____

Section IV

SUMMARY

I have reviewed the clinical privileges requested and my recommendation concerning the specific clinical privileges requested is as follows:

❏ I recommend granting all privileges as requested by the applicant.

❏ I recommend granting privileges as requested by the applicant with the limitations specified below:*

❏ I recommend not granting the applicant the privileges listed below:*

❏ I recommend not granting any privileges requested by the applicant:*

*Please explain any reservations or concerns regarding any specific privilege/services requested by the applicant.

_____

_____

_____

_____

FIGURE 1.1
PROFESSIONAL REFERENCE QUESTIONNAIRE (CONT.)

I have reviewed this practitioner's application for appointment/affiliation and my recommendation concerning this practitioner's application for appointment/affiliation is as follows:

❏ I recommend the applicant.

❏ I recommend the applicant with the reservations listed below:**

❏ I do not recommend the applicant. **

**Please explain any reservations or concerns regarding the applicant's request for appointment/affiliation.

_____

_____

_____

_____

Please use this section for any additional comments, information, or recommendations that may be relevant to our decision to grant appointment/affiliation or specific clinical privileges/services to the applicant.

_____

_____

_____

_____

If you would like to discuss this applicant with someone from our organization, please call _____

at _____ and a mutually convenient time for a phone conversation will be arranged.

Reference provided by: _____

Signature: _____ **Date:** _____ **Field of practice:** _____

Telephone: (_____) _____ **ext.**_____ **E-mail:** _____

Evergreen or "Forevermore" Evaluations

As noted above, an important part of initial competence verification is obtaining a clinical evaluation from the department chair at a hospital or university where the practitioner practiced. Often, when MSPs attempt to obtain this evaluation, the individual who was in that role while the practitioner held privileges there is no longer in that role, and the new department chair is unable to attest to the individual's competence or prior performance. One way to ensure that your organization is able to disclose thorough credentialing and competence information to other organizations is to complete evergreen (also commonly referred to as "forevermore") evaluations when a practitioner leaves your organization.

An evergreen evaluation incorporates the affiliation verification and clinical evaluation into one form. For the affiliation verification, your medical staff services department can complete:

- The practitioner's dates of affiliation at your organization

- The department that the practitioner was assigned to

- Staff category (e.g., active, affiliate, associate, etc.)

- Privileges the practitioner held at your organization

- Recent utilization history/volume (e.g., case logs)

If the practitioner had no disclosable actions, include a statement that indicates that while the individual was on staff, he or she met all requirements of staff membership and had no clinical or other performance concerns. See the "Common Missteps" section at the end of this chapter if the practitioner has disclosable actions, such as restrictions to privileges, sanctions, or disciplinary action.

For the clinical evaluation section of the evergreen verification, the organization should include a statement at the beginning of the form that indicates that the evaluation is being completed on X date by the current department chair. The statement should indicate that the information is valid through that date and is a representation of the individual's performance only while affiliated with your organization.

The current department chair should complete the clinical evaluation section to the best of his or her knowledge. The questions should be the same questions that the organization uses on its clinical evaluation forms (and others if deemed appropriate by the organization), and you can elect to incorporate the six general competencies to ensure the evaluation is meaningful. You want to ensure that the department chair signs and dates the evaluation.

In the instance of practitioners who have had formal disciplinary actions and/or have been under a formal investigation, medical staff leaders may wish to consider whether the evergreen letter will be used as a response. Some organizations have determined that in these instances, they will respond only to the specific questions asked from the requesting facility (See the "Common Missteps" section at the end of this chapter for more information.) Still other organizations create a specific response given the circumstances of the practitioner's departure. It is important for organizations to develop a routine procedure for responding to queries regarding practitioners with less than stellar performance. The routine procedure, along with the content of the responses on the individual practitioner, should be determined following the input of legal counsel.

Competence Assessment Through FPPE After Granting Clinical Privileges

Once an applicant has been granted clinical privileges by the board of directors, or after he or she has been granted temporary privileges (see Chapter 3 for verifying competence prior to granting temporary privileges), the organization should monitor the practitioner's competence through an initial assessment. For Joint Commission–accredited organizations, FPPE is required to assess the individual's ability to competently exercise clinical privileges using your staff, equipment, and resources. For non-Joint Commission–accredited organizations, initial competence assessment should be incorporated as best practice to ensure safe, quality patient care.

In addition to each of the department chairs, the organization's credentials committee plays a significant role in determining what the initial competence assessment or FPPE should entail. We discussed the option to offer precepting if an applicant does not have enough current clinical competence and needs to gain additional training and experience to demonstrate current clinical competence. Some additional examples of initial competence assessment options are listed below:

- Core privileges: The credentials committee could indicate that all department chairs must assign a minimum number of retrospective chart reviews for core privileges. The department chair would have the option to increase the number of chart reviews, but it could not fall below the minimum set by the credentials committee. For example, if the credentials committee determines that all departments should have a minimum of 10 retrospective chart reviews for core privileges, a department chair may decide that for his or her department, 10 is too few. The department chair could set the initial FPPE criteria higher, such as 20 retrospective chart reviews for all core privileges and direct observation for five patients with a specific diagnosis. It is important to note, however, that the cases need to be a full representation of all privileges included in the core. For example, the proctor could not conduct retrospective chart review of 10 patients with a similar diagnosis as this would not be a representation of everything included in the core.

- Special procedures: For more invasive or specialized procedures or more acute patients, the department chair should carefully consider what type of initial competence assessment is appropriate. This often involves direct observation for a specified number of procedures to demonstrate competence prior to allowing the practitioner to practice independently. For example, if your organization has the Da Vinci robot, there are competence requirements that must be submitted prior to granting privileges to use this equipment (i.e., completion of appropriate training, etc.). However, initial competence assessment at your organization may include direct observation for a specified number of cases.

- Additional requirements: As mentioned earlier in this chapter, if an applicant does not have recent experience relevant to the privileges he or she has requested, the department chair has the option of adding requirements to the FPPE to better evaluate the practitioner's current clinical competence. For example, if the minimum criteria for core privileges in a department is 10 retrospective reviews for most applicants and the applicant does not have recent experience, the department chair could increase the FPPE requirement either in volume or by adding requirements, such as direct observation, precepting, or remedial courses.

The most important thing for department chairs to remember when developing FPPE plans is to customize the plans as needed for each individual. The department chair typically assigns the oversight or proctoring of a new practitioner to a tenured member of the department with similar privileges. Anyone assigned as a proctor must hold current clinical privileges equivalent to those that they are proctoring. After completing the proctoring (or earlier, should an issue arise), the evaluations and recommendations from the proctor are forwarded to the department chair for final review. The department chair should then make a recommendation to the credentials committee to decide whether the FPPE was successfully completed or if additional monitoring/proctoring is required. For example, if the FPPE included retrospective chart reviews, and the proctor indicated that there were documentation concerns noted, the department chair may recommend that the practitioner attend documentation training specific to the organization and assign additional retrospective reviews to ensure that his or her performance improves.

If the initial FPPE indicates that there are significant clinical care concerns, the department chair must determine what the appropriate next steps are to address these concerns. The organization should keep in mind, however, that if the action taken to address the concern involves any corrective action, it must follow the medical staff bylaws to determine whether the practitioner is entitled to due process. For example, if the department chair recommends limiting the practitioner's privileges to perform certain procedures, a limitation of privileges for competence concerns would typically entitle the individual to due process, and if limited for more than 30 days, it is reportable to the state board and NPDB.

Additionally, organizations need to also consider that recommendations for prospective proctoring may be reportable. Prospective proctoring that requires preauthorization (when the proctor is required to approve a practitioner's plan of care prior to treating a patient or prior to care being delivered) is reportable to the NPDB.

Common Missteps

The following are common missteps during initial credentialing:

- **Affiliation verification versus clinical evaluation:** Often, organizations combine the affiliation verification and a clinical evaluation into one form; however, it is more likely that they will get a quicker and more accurate response if they separate these two forms. The affiliation verification is typically sent to the medical staff services department at all current or prior hospitals where the practitioner held or currently holds clinical privileges and is completed by the MSP, as the keeper of the credentialing database. MSPs can verify dates of affiliation, staff status, type of privileges held, and whether there were any performance or quality concerns. MSPs should not answer questions pertaining to the practitioner's competence or make recommendations specific to the practitioner's request for privileges at the new organization. Rather, these tasks should be deferred to the appropriate department chair or peer references. Keeping these two forms separate helps expedite the process and ensures that your organization receives the information in a more timely manner. If you combine them, MSPs may complete the section that they are qualified to complete and return the rest of the form incomplete, as they are not qualified to answer the evaluation questions. As noted in the "Evergreen or 'Forevermore' Evaluations" section earlier in this chapter, it is efficient to combine the two when a practitioner leaves the organization, as the information will not change.

- **Failure to ask the right questions on the medical staff application:** This is one of the most common pitfalls in credentialing. It is difficult to draft questions that cover any and all situations that should be disclosed by the applicant; however, organizations should attempt to be as thorough as possible. For example, asking if an applicant has ever been the subject of "formal disciplinary action" at any healthcare institution is rather vague. The applicant may not consider certain actions to be formal disciplinary action, and, therefore, based on the way the question is worded, he or she may not disclose pertinent information. For example, perhaps he or she was under investigation or had numerous incident reports filed against him or her that were handled at the department level through collegial intervention. Because these actions are not considered formal corrective or disciplinary action through the MEC, the applicant may not feel that he or she needs to disclose the information. However, if the application specifically asks whether the applicant has ever been the subject of any current, former, or pending complaints; the subject of a current or pending investigation or formal review; or placed on probation, suspended, reprimanded, or received any other type of disciplinary or corrective action—the applicant would be required to disclose that information.

- **Questions on affiliation verifications:** Ensuring that the questions on your affiliation verifications are thorough is just as important as ensuring that questions on your application are thorough to ensure that other organizations disclose all relevant information regarding the applicant. After receiving an affiliation verification, organizations must carefully read the questions and respond accordingly (always, of course, ensuring that the appropriate third-party form that authorizes the release of the information in good faith and releases all parties from liability in doing so, is signed by the applicant). An organization will not (and should not) disclose specific actions if the questionnaire does not ask for it. An organization must disclose information in good faith, and disclosing more than what is requested may leave the organization vulnerable to certain liabilities. For example, if an affiliation verification form asks whether there has been any disciplinary action *taken* against the practitioner in question, the organization may not disclose a *pending* action. Therefore, your organization should ask whether there have been any disciplinary actions or whether there are any impending reviews or investigations. A common mistake at the time of recredentialing is for an organization to include questions that start with, "In the past two years …." Just because you received an initial verification two years ago with no disclosures does not mean that something wasn't missed. For example, perhaps two years ago, the organization's policy was not to disclose certain actions to other hospitals, but the policy has changed. If the action occurred more than two years ago, they would not be obligated to disclose the information if your question is limited to the past two years.

 The Medical Staff's Guide to Overcoming Competence Assessment Challenges

- **Inadequate review of red flags:** When an MSP or medical staff leader identifies a red flag (something in the applicant's practice history that appears abnormal, such as not completing a residency program in the normal time frame, an excessive number of prior malpractice claims, significant gaps in work history, etc.), the organization should ensure that it thoroughly investigates the concern. Ensuring that all discrepancies or concerns that are noted during the credentialing process are thoroughly reviewed and followed up on is an essential part of the MSP's role.

- **Failure to thoroughly review submitted verifications:** MSPs should also closely review the responses they receive from peer references, other healthcare institutions, licensing agencies, and training programs. They need to compare the dates provided from the applicant to the dates provided by the source for discrepancies. They also need to evaluate whether the organization answered all questions thoroughly on the verification form and flag any concerns for the department chair to review. If the organization did not complete the verification form and instead provided a generalized or template response, the MSP should verify that the response includes a statement that confirms that the applicant was not the subject of formal disciplinary action or complaints and that there were no quality concerns. If the organization does not provide this information to the MSP, the MSP should put the responsibility of obtaining a clear and thorough response back on the applicant.

In summary, initial competence assessment goes above and beyond the initial credentialing process. Organizations have many different options to not only ensure that new practitioners are clinically competent to perform the privileges requested, but to also ensure that they maintain competence through precepting or initial proctoring.

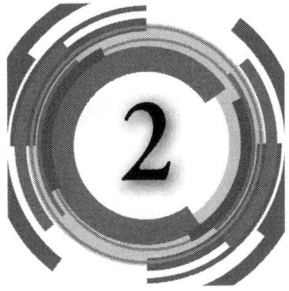

2 Assessing Competence in the Ambulatory Setting

Carol S. Cairns, CPMSM, CPCS

CASE STUDY

Mary Barr, CPMSM, was new to her position as director of medical affairs at St. John Medical Center. With extensive experience as a medical services professional (MSP), Mary initially focused her attention on the scope of credentialing and privileging of current medical staff members, advanced practice professionals, and new applicants. As the months passed, Mary realized that only some of the physicians working at the four St. John Family Healthcare Centers had privileges at St. John Medical Center. Further, the scope of the privileges granted to these physicians was silent regarding their practice at the health centers.

When Mary asked the vice president of medical affairs (VPMA), he informed her that there was no need to privilege any of the practitioners for their work at the family health centers. The VPMA stated that because these practitioners were employees of the medical center, he felt the human resources process was sufficient. Therefore, no site-specific privileging process was required. To support this view, the VPMA cited the organization's recent Joint Commission survey along with two previous surveys since the establishment of these health centers. The VPMA indicated that The Joint Commission raised no issues.

What should Mary's next steps be? Should Mary drop the issue given she has plenty of responsibilities needing her attention, or should she pursue the issue further? If she pursues the issue, how should Mary proceed?

Understanding Healthcare Delivery in Ambulatory Settings

Healthcare organizations have become increasingly complex. In past decades, most organizations provided patient care within the walls of the facility. Essentially, no clinical care was provided outside the facility, but this care delivery model is no longer the norm—quite the contrary!

Many healthcare organizations and/or systems provide significant healthcare services outside the four walls of the hospital. There are many hospital- or system-owned ambulatory care facilities and services. Examples include:

- Cancer care centers

- Birthing centers

- Outpatient surgery centers

- Outpatient testing facilities

- Radiology or radiation therapy units

- Rehabilitation, physical, and occupational therapy services

In addition, hospitals and/or systems may also own a variety of practice locations where practitioners provide care. The practitioners within these facilities may be employees of the hospital or under contract to provide services. Some examples are:

- Individual practitioner offices

    - Primary care (e.g., family medicine, internal medicine, pediatrics, etc.)

    - Specialist care (e.g., plastic surgery, gastroenterology, dermatology, oral maxillofacial surgery, etc.)

- Multiple practitioners in a group setting

    - Family care centers

    - Single-specialty group practices

    - Multispecialty group practices

    - Behavioral health counseling centers

    - Maternity care facilities

The Medical Staff's Guide to Overcoming Competence Assessment Challenges

- Complementary and/or alternative care services

- Comprehensive pain centers

- Urgent care centers

- Wound care facilities (with or without hyperbaric chambers)

Often, these sites of care bear the name of the parent organization. In the case study described at the beginning of this chapter, the ancillary practices are called St. John Family Healthcare Centers. Another indicator of the relationship between the hospital and the service is whether the patient records belong to the physician or to the hospital. For example, if the physician leaves the community, who retains the patients' records?

The care rendered at these hospital-owned sites may be provided by the following types of practitioners:

- Physicians

- Dentists

- Oral surgeons

- Podiatrists

- Psychiatrists

- Psychologists

- Physician assistants (PA)

- Advanced practice nurses

  - Nurse practitioners (NP)

  - Nurse anesthetists

  - Nurse midwives

  - Clinical nurse specialists

Requirements of Regulators and Accreditation Agencies

The Centers for Medicare & Medicaid Services (CMS)'s requirements for privileging make no distinction between the previously mentioned practitioners. For example, CMS requires hospitals to apply the same medical staff privileging process to all practitioners regardless of whether they are physicians, PAs, or NPs. This privileging process applies whether a practitioner is under contract with the hospital, employed by the hospital, or independent of the organization.

Key to the decision to privilege or not to privilege is whether the practitioner provides a "medical level of care." In general, this language pertains to practitioners who—in accordance with state licensure regulations and organizational policy—can order diagnostic and/or therapeutic tests or modalities, perform procedures generally done by physicians, or have been authorized to perform history and physical examinations (with or without being countersigned by a physician).

Practitioners who do not provide a medical level of care do not need to be privileged. For example, if a nurse practitioner is functioning as a nurse, case manager, infection control nurse, or manager of a care unit at the site, the medical staff does not have to privilege him or her. The term medical level of care applies to individuals providing a higher level of clinical services. CMS uses this term to differentiate the level of medical care that physicians and surgeons provide from nurses, laboratory technologists, radiology technicians, etc., who may also work at these ambulatory sites.

The best indicator of the hospital's need to credential and privilege practitioners providing a medical level of care at the external site is the CMS certification number (CCN). If the hospital and the site or sites in question all have the same CCN and bill a facility fee for the services rendered, then CMS considers the site part of the hospital. Thus, the site is subjected to the same credentialing and privileging processes that apply to practitioners who are privileged to provide care at the hospital.

Clarification: CCN stands for CMS certification number. The CCN verifies that the practitioner has been Medicare certified and for what type of services. The CCN is also referred to as the national provider identifier, the Medicare/Medicaid provider number, or simply "provider number."

The Joint Commission also requires facilities to privilege practitioners for care provided in the hospital-owned ambulatory setting. Inclusion of the ambulatory site(s) is addressed in the introductory portions of the *Comprehensive Accreditation Manual for Hospitals*. If your hospital is accredited by another organization, double-check its privileging requirements for ambulatory sites.

Thus, the old response, "If the service does not happen within our walls, we are not responsible," is clearly no longer accurate.

Scope of Privileges at the Ambulatory Site

Once the hospital has established which sites require practitioners to be privileged, the medical staff needs to evaluate the scope of services provided at the site by physicians and advanced practice professionals (APP), such as NPs and PAs. Thereafter, the medical staff delineates site-specific privileges and commensurate criteria.

For example, the scope of privileges defined for an office-based family practitioner would differ from a family practitioner in an urgent care center or birthing center. The office-based physician could potentially be caring for patients of all ages and may or may not do minor procedures. The physician at the urgent care center would generally be treating minor injuries and illnesses and not be providing preventive medicine, such as immunizations, Pap smears, or smoking cessation counseling. The family practitioner practicing at the birthing center would only need privileges related to obstetrics and newborn care.

Examples of ambulatory privileges versus acute care privileges are:

- The family practitioner may not treat any pediatric or newborn patients in the hospital but may see this patient population in the office setting.

- The family practitioner or internal medicine specialist may not do Pap smears, proctology examinations, vasectomies, or joint injections in the acute care setting but may elect to perform these procedures in the ambulatory site.

- The physician providing care in the urgent care center may be allowed to suture lacerations but may not meet the minimum criteria to do so in the hospital's emergency department.

Once the care provided in the various hospital-owned ambulatory sites has been defined, the medical staff has several options for designing the privilege delineation form. The options might include:

- If the privileges and eligibility criteria already described in the hospital privilege form match the privileges for the ambulatory site, the organization could simply add the additional site(s) of care to the existing privilege form.

- If the privileges and eligibility criteria are very similar and essentially cover the same practitioners, the organization may simply add language such as "office-based practice" and identify the privileges/procedures that would apply in that setting only.

- Create an ambulatory site privilege form specific to the clinical practice at that site. This would need to be done for any practitioner who did not practice in the acute care setting.

Figure 2.1 is an example of an office-based family medicine or internal medicine core privilege delineation form.

Figure 2.2 is an example of privilege delineation language for an ambulatory center subspecialist in pediatric endocrinology. This privilege description could be added to the organization's inpatient pediatric endocrinology privilege form or utilized only for the ambulatory site as depicted in Figure 2.1 for family practice.

It is important to recognize that privilege delineation is also required for APPs who provide care in the ambulatory setting. To keep the process of privilege delineation simple, we recommend adapting the current methodology for delineating privileges for the hospital setting to the ambulatory setting—recognizing the delineation must be specific for the advanced practice registered nurse or PA qualifications and scope of care. This delineation should also clearly state any applicable supervision, collaboration, or consultation required by a physician.

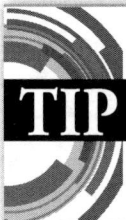

> **TIP**
>
> For those organizations using a core or criteria-based privileging system, creating language specific for the ambulatory setting is relatively easy. Simply evaluate the current language for the acute care setting and modify it for the new practice setting. Then determine the applicable procedures to be included in the core and those that should be identified separately with applicable eligibility criteria.

Responsibility for Privileging in an Ambulatory Setting

If the healthcare facility determines that the ambulatory site(s) fall under the responsibility of the hospital (see "Requirements of Regulators and Accreditation Agencies" above), the medical staff is responsible for delineating privileges in the various nonacute settings. Thus, the current department chair would evaluate the privileges requested by the applicant and provide input or recommendations to the credentials committee. Subsequently, the credentials committee's recommendation is forwarded to the medical executive

> **FIGURE 2.1**
>
> **AMBULATORY CLINICAL PRIVILEGES REQUEST FORM**
> **(FAMILY MEDICINE OR INTERNAL MEDICINE)**

Name: Effective from __/__/__ to __/__/__

[] Initial Appointment

[] Reappointment

Note: If any scope of practice is covered by an exclusive contractual agreement, practitioners who are not a party to the agreement are not eligible to request the scope of practice, regardless of education, training, and experience. Exclusive contracts are indicated by [EC].

All new applicants must meet the following requirements as approved by the board of directors, effective __/__/__.

To be eligible to apply for ambulatory clinical core privileges, the applicant must meet the following criteria:

- Successful completion of an Accreditation Council for Graduate Medical Education (ACGME) or American Osteopathic Association (AOA)–accredited postgraduate training program in family medicine or internal medicine

- Current certification or active participation in the examination process leading to board certification in family practice by the American Board of Family Practice or the American Osteopathic Board of Family Physicians or by the American Board of Internal Medicine or the American Osteopathic Board of Internal Medicine

- Applicants for initial appointment must be able to demonstrate active clinical part-time practice within the past 12 months

And

To be eligible to renew ambulatory clinical core privileges, the applicant must meet the following renewal of privileges criteria:

- Current demonstrated competence and an active clinical part-time practice with acceptable results in the privileges requested for the past 24 months based on results of quality assessment/improvement activities and outcomes. Evidence of current ability to perform privileges requested is required of all applicants for renewal of privileges.

- Maintenance of certification.

Applicant: Check off the "Requested" box for each privilege requested. New applicants may be requested to provide documentation of the number and types of outpatient cases during the past 24 months. Applicants have the burden of producing information deemed adequate by the [hospital/clinic] for a proper evaluation of current competence and other qualifications and for resolving any doubts.

Department chair/chief: Check the appropriate box for recommendation on the last page of this form. If you choose not to recommend the applicant or recommend with a condition, provide the condition or explanation on the last page of this form.

FIGURE 2.1

AMBULATORY CLINICAL PRIVILEGES REQUEST FORM
(FAMILY MEDICINE OR INTERNAL MEDICINE) (CONT.)

Ambulatory (Family Medicine or Internal Medicine) Core Privileges:

[] Requested: Evaluate, diagnose, and treat pediatric and adult patients for common illnesses and injuries in the ambulatory setting. Privileges include but are not limited to:

- Suture uncomplicated lacerations

- Treat burns, superficial and partial thickness

- Drain abscesses

- Interpret EKGs

- Provide local anesthetic

- Manage uncomplicated minor closed fractures and uncomplicated dislocations

- Perform simple skin biopsy or excisions

- Remove nonpenetrating corneal foreign body

Arthrocentesis:

[] Requested: Successful completion of an ACGME or AOA residency training program in family medicine or internal medicine in the past 12 months. Applicants must provide evidence that the training program included arthrocentesis or demonstrate required previous experience (at least [n] procedures in the past 12 months).

Renewal of privileges: Demonstrated current competence and evidence of the performance of at least [n] procedures in the past 24 months.

Acknowledgement of Practitioner

I have requested only those privileges for which by education, training, current experience, and demonstrated performance I am qualified to perform and for which I wish to exercise at _____, and I understand that:

- (a) In exercising any clinical privileges granted, I am constrained by the hospital and medical staff policies and rules applicable generally and any applicable to the particular situation.

- (b) Any restriction on the clinical privileges granted to me is waived in an emergency situation and, in such situation, my actions are governed by the applicable section of the medical staff bylaws or related documents.

Signed: Date:

          The Medical Staff's Guide to Overcoming Competence Assessment Challenges

---

FIGURE 2.1

AMBULATORY CLINICAL PRIVILEGES REQUEST FORM (FAMILY MEDICINE OR INTERNAL MEDICINE) (CONT.)

Division Director/Department Chair's Recommendation

I have reviewed the requested clinical privileges and supporting documentation for the above-named applicant and make the following recommendation(s):

[] Recommend all requested privileges

[] Recommend privileges with the following conditions/modifications:

[] Do not recommend the following requested privileges:

Privilege   Condition/modification/explanation

1.

2.

3.

4.

Notes:

Department Chief Signature: Date:

********** For Medical Staff Office Use Only **********

Credentials Committee Action: Date:

Medical Executive Committee Action: Date:

Board of Directors Action: Date:

FIGURE 2.2

AMBULATORY PEDIATRIC ENDOCRINOLOGY CORE PRIVILEGES

Requested   Evaluate, diagnose, consult, and provide treatment to infants, children, and adolescents with diseases or disorders resulting from an abnormality in the endocrine glands, including but not limited to diabetes mellitus, growth failure, unusual size for age, early or late pubertal development, birth defects, the genital region, and disorders of the thyroid, adrenal, and pituitary glands. Ambulatory core privileges in this specialty include the procedures on the attached procedure list[1] and such other procedures that are extensions of the same techniques and skills.

---

[1]The form would then detail non-core procedures from core procedures as exemplified in the family medicine form.

---

committee (MEC), which provides a recommendation to the governing body. The governing body then makes decisions based on the recommendation.

However, in some organizations, medical staff leaders are reluctant to expand the scope of their responsibility to include hospital-owned clinics and employed physicians. Also, because some practitioners provide care only in the ambulatory setting, the designated medical staff leader may have no firsthand knowledge of the practitioner or his or her competence. Some of these practitioners may have only membership (but no privileges) in the acute care setting.

To solve this challenge, some organizations have created a separate committee or department that assumes responsibility for credentialing, privileging, and competence assessment for practitioners working in ambulatory sites. Some organizations have designated a medical staff ambulatory services department, defined medical staff leadership selection methodologies, and outlined specific responsibilities and reporting structures. Depending on the referral base and culture of the organization, some facilities have created a seat on the MEC to represent employed, contracted, and independent practitioners in the ambulatory setting.

Medical Staff Category Versus Privileges

If a practitioner is actively caring for patients in the hospital as well as the ambulatory setting, he or she probably belongs in the active staff category. However, for those practitioners who solely practice at the urgent care center, office, or diagnostic center, what staff category applies?

Organizations must first separate the concepts of membership and privileges. These are two distinct terms. Membership refers to the practitioner's rights and responsibilities on the medical staff, such as the whether the practitioner has the right to vote or serve as an officer. The term "privileges" refers only to what clinical activity the practitioner requests and the governing board grants. Thus, a physician could be office-based only and never care for a patient in the hospital but refer all patient diagnostic testing and admissions to the hospital. In this case, some organizations would see value in appointing this physician to the active medical staff category with all the same rights and responsibilities of physicians who routinely care for inpatients. The relationship with the physician is beneficial to the hospital, so the hospital wants to reward him or her with the right to serve in office and vote on medical staff matters.

Other organizations may choose to create a different category for practitioners who are not actively practicing within the acute care setting. A common term for this category is affiliate staff. The affiliate staff category may be reserved for practitioners who maintain a clinical practice in the hospital service area and wish to be able to follow their patients when they are admitted to the hospital. These members may do the following:

- Order noninvasive outpatient diagnostic tests and services

- Visit patients in the hospital

- Review medical records

- Attend medical staff or department/service meetings, continuing medical education functions, and social events

These practitioners generally do not have authorization to exercise any clinical privileges within the hospital and may or may not vote on medical staff affairs or hold office, depending on the medical staff's culture. Members of this category fulfill or comply with any applicable medical staff or hospital policies and procedures.

Competence Assessment in the Ambulatory Setting

Essentially, assessing competence in the ambulatory setting does not differ from the processes used in the acute care setting. The same requirements and expectations outlined throughout this book are applied to the ambulatory setting as well. It does not matter what terms the medical staff and organization use to describe the competence assessment function, the process will be the same. (Common terms applied to the function may include performance monitoring, performance improvement, quality assessment, quality improvement, ongoing professional practice evaluation [OPPE]/focused professional practice evaluation [FPPE], peer review, etc.)

Terminology for competence assessment varies by the regulating body (CMS) and the accrediting agency (The Joint Commission, Healthcare Facilities Accreditation Program, Det Norske Veritas [DNV], Accreditation Association for Ambulatory Health Care, etc.). Organizations must adhere to the requirements of the applicable accrediting body.

If the accrediting body is the same for the acute care and ambulatory settings, the competence assessment processes should be the same—just modified to the site of care. The facility may choose to apply some measurement indicators and benchmark rates to all settings, such as those reflecting professionalism, communication skills, or patient satisfaction. Others will be different and reflect the specific skills needed and procedures performed in the various settings.

For example, the inpatient facility may assess a practitioner's competence using mortality, blood usage, and patient length of stay as competence indicators. In the office-based setting, the organization may choose to monitor immunization rates, blood sugar monitoring for diabetic patients, and colon cancer screening for patients older than age 50. The indicators for measurement may be different in the ambulatory setting and the acute care setting, but the process should essentially mirror the medical staff process as outlined within the medical staff bylaws, policies and procedures, and performance improvement plan.

Figure 2.3 provides some examples of physician indicators of performance that apply to the ambulatory setting. The Six General Competencies adapted from the Accreditation Council for Graduate Medical Education (ACGME) and the American Board of Medical Specialties (ABMS) joint initiative serve as the framework for categorizing the measurement indicator (See Chapter 1 for a full list of the six core competencies).

Note that the measurements also include benchmark targets (acceptable and excellent). Setting two targets allows the medical staff and practitioner to have a clear understanding of performance that is below expectation, performance that meets expectation, and performance that exceeds the expectation. Using two targets for benchmarking avoids the "pass/fail" concept inherent when only one target is established.

FIGURE 2.3
PHYSICIAN INDICATORS OF PERFORMANCE

Competency	Specialty	Indicator		Acceptable Target	Excellence Target
Medical Clinical Knowledge	FP, IM, OB-Gyne	Diabetes - LDL-C screening performed	rate	75%	100%
Medical Clinical Knowledge	Ophthalmology	Dilated macular or fundus exam performed with documentation of the level of severity of retinopathy and the presence or absence of macular edema during one or more visits in the past 12 months in patients with a diagnosis of diabetic retinopathy	rate	75%	95%
Systems-based Practice	All	NPSG - Handwashing	rule	3	1
Interpersonal and communication skills	All	Medical records compliance—office charts completed within 1 day	rate	75%	95%
Professionalism	All	Validated incidents of inappropriate behavior	rule	2	0
Interpersonal and communication skills	All	Office survey regarding practitioner took time to answer my questions	rate	50th percentile	90th percentile

For example, in Figure 2.3, the "average" benchmark rate for performing diabetic screening is 75%. To be considered "excellent," the benchmark is 100%. If only one target is used (e.g., 75%), practitioners either pass or fail this standard. Setting two targets promotes "raising the bar," since "average" is considered acceptable, and for most practitioners being rated as "average" is not sufficient. Therefore, most practitioners would strive to improve their compliance with the practice standard. This effort then raises the overall standard of care.

Further, falling below the target of 75% clearly notifies the practitioner that his or her performance is below the acceptable standard. These data would also be evaluated by medical staff leadership to determine whether there were performance issues that needed to be addressed.

Assessing the Competence of APPs in the Ambulatory Setting

It is important for healthcare organizations to monitor not only the performance of physicians in the ambulatory settings but also the performance of APPs. Quite often, the monitoring indicators are similar, if not the same, for APPs and physicians.

To help organizations define performance indicators for PAs, the American Academy of Physician Assistants (AAPA) has prepared and published a document entitled *Physician Assistant Competency Measures*. The AAPA has given permission for this document to be included in its entirety in this book (see Figure 2.4). The first two pages of the competence measurements are basic and apply to all PAs, regardless of specialty. The third page reflects specialty-specific competencies for a PA specializing in orthopedics and pertains to the privileges delineated. The final page contains the sign-off and comments from for the evaluator.

Once again, the framework utilized by the AAPA in developing this form is that of the ACGME and ABMS six general competencies. This comprehensive form outlines competencies that apply not only to the office setting but also to the acute care setting.

Physician Assistant Competency Measures also provides another way of benchmarking. The organization would simply establish a level of expected performance utilizing the numerical (1–5) rating scale.

This document also provides many examples of performance expectations that would apply not only to PAs but also to physicians, podiatrists, NPs, nurse midwives, and other practitioners.

FIGURE 2.4
PHYSICIAN ASSISTANT COMPETENCY MEASURES

Competency Measure Note: A score of 1 or 2 requires comment in the space provided.	Unacceptable Clearly inadequate; requires remediation	Poor Many deficiencies	Satisfactory Adequate	Very Good Exceeds in many areas- top 20%	Excellent Superior in every way- top 10%
Patient Care (and Procedures)					
• History taking: accurate and complete	1	2	3	4	5
• Physical exam: required components present	1	2	3	4	5
• Complete assessment and plans	1	2	3	4	5
• Provides quality patient education	1	2	3	4	5
• Competently performs medical and surgical procedures delineated by medical staff privileges–overall evaluation (See page 3 for department specific privilege, focused evaluations.)	1	2	3	4	5
Medical Knowledge					
• Appropriate selection of diagnostic tests	1	2	3	4	5
• Appropriate interpretation/analysis of test results	1	2	3	4	5
• Appropriate integration of history and physical findings and diagnostic studies to formulate a differential diagnosis.	1	2	3	4	5
• Overall integration of clinical information into treatment planning	1	2	3	4	5
• Pharmacological knowledge/ appropriate ordering of therapeutics	1	2	3	4	5
Practice-Based Learning and Improvement					
• Applies evidence-based medicine to clinical decisions	1	2	3	4	5
• Awareness of quality improvement measures and application to clinical practice	1	2	3	4	5
• Facilitates the learning of students and other health care professionals	1	2	3	4	5

PA Name: _____   Date of Evaluation: _____

American Academy of PHYSICIAN ASSISTANTS

© 2013 American Academy of Physician Assistants — page 1

FIGURE 2.4

PHYSICIAN ASSISTANT COMPETENCY MEASURES (CONT.)

Competency Measure Note: A score of 1 or 2 requires comment in the space provided.	Unacceptable Clearly inadequate; requires remediation	Poor Many deficiencies	Satisfactory Adequate	Very Good Exceeds in many areas- top 20%	Excellent Superior in every way- top 10%
Professionalism					
Displays sensitivity and responsiveness to patients' culture, age, gender, and disabilities	1	2	3	4	5
Understanding of the legal and regulatory requirements governing PA practice and the role of the PA.	1	2	3	4	5
Commitment to personal excellence and ongoing professional development.	1	2	3	4	5
Interpersonal & Communication Skills					
Communications and behaviors with patients are effective and appropriate.	1	2	3	4	5
Communications and behaviors with physician supervisors are effective and appropriate.	1	2	3	4	5
Demonstrates emotional resilience and stability, adaptability, flexibility and tolerance of ambiguity and anxiety	1	2	3	4	5
Uses effective listening, nonverbal, explanatory, interviewing and writing skills to elicit and provide information.	1	2	3	4	5
Systems Based Practice					
Uses information technology resources to support patient care decisions and patient education.	1	2	3	4	5
Practices cost-effective health care and resources allocation that does not compromise quality of care.	1	2	3	4	5
Applies medical information and clinical data systems to provide more effective, efficient patient care.	1	2	3	4	5

PA Name: _____   Date of Evaluation: _____

American Academy of
PHYSICIAN ASSISTANTS

© 2013 American Academy of Physician Assistants — page 2

The Medical Staff's Guide to Overcoming Competence Assessment Challenges

FIGURE 2.4
PHYSICIAN ASSISTANT COMPETENCY MEASURES (CONT.)

Competency Measure–Orthopaedics

Note: A score of 1 or 2 requires comment in the space provided.

Competency Measure	Unacceptable — Clearly inadequate; requires remediation	Poor — Many deficiencies	Satisfactory — Adequate	Very Good — Exceeds in many areas - top 20%	Excellent — Superior in every way - top 10%
X-ray Interpretation:					
Demonstrates accurate interpretation of findings	1	2	3	4	5
Provides complete documentation	1	2	3	4	5
Fracture/dislocation reduction:					
Demonstrates appropriate technique	1	2	3	4	5
Achieves acceptable alignment	1	2	3	4	5
Provides appropriate post-reduction management/immobilization	1	2	3	4	5
Cast/Splint Application					
Demonstrates appropriate technique	1	2	3	4	5
Applies appropriate splint type and selects appropriate materials	1	2	3	4	5
Assistant at Surgery					
Maintains sterile technique	1	2	3	4	5
Demonstrates appropriate patient positioning/draping	1	2	3	4	5
Provides effective retraction/exposure	1	2	3	4	5
Demonstrates acceptable wound closure techniques, including approximation of layers, selection of closure material, and dressing application	1	2	3	4	5
Medical Management					
Antibiotics ordered appropriately (1 hour prior to surgery, stopped in 24 hours post-op, appropriate drug selected)	1	2	3	4	5
DVT prophylaxis ordered appropriately	1	2	3	4	5
Pain management appropriate	1	2	3	4	5

American Academy of PHYSICIAN ASSISTANTS

PA Name: _____   Date of Evaluation: _____

© 2013 American Academy of Physician Assistants — page 3

FIGURE 2.4
PHYSICIAN ASSISTANT COMPETENCY MEASURES (CONT.)

Evaluator Level of Interaction:

☐ Minimum-occasional encounters
☐ Moderate-weekly encounters
☐ Extensive-daily encounters

Evaluator

☐ Physician (MD/DO)
☐ Peer (PA)

Comments: (Required for any Rating of "1" or "2")

Evaluator Signature: _____

Date of Evaluation: _____

Evaluator Name: _____

PA Name: _____

© 2013 American Academy of Physician Assistants — page 4

The Medical Staff's Guide to Overcoming Competence Assessment Challenges

Revisiting St. John Medical Center

Now that we understand how to assess practitioner competence within the ambulatory setting, let's revisit our case study. The medical staff leaders of St. John Medical Center and the VPMA are daunted by the enormity of the task ahead of them. Sensing they were overwhelmed by what needed to be done, Mary, the MSP, created a simple five-step plan to focus the organization's attention on the path ahead. This plan outlines a reasonable approach to ensuring the competence of the practitioners at the four St. John Family Healthcare Centers.

Step 1: Determine the settings of care and the practitioners within each setting that need to be privileged by St. John Medical Center.

Step 2: Evaluate the requirements of the applicable regulator and/or accrediting agency. Determine whether there is a requirement for site-specific privileging. If not, also determine the risk to patient care if these practitioners are not privileged and thus their competence is not assessed.

Step 3: Determine the scope of care provided by each practitioner at each ambulatory site. Develop a site-specific privilege delineation system that avoids duplication of efforts with the existing methodology used for the acute care setting.

Step 4: Evaluate the differences and similarities of the ambulatory service and hospital. Determine the simplest but most appropriate route to integrate credentialing, privileging, and competence assessment responsibilities within the medical center and medical staff structure. Assign responsibility for these functions.

Step 5: Create meaningful competence assessment tools for the specific site(s) of care and monitor the performance of all applicable practitioners on an ongoing basis. Review the data on a periodic basis and provide feedback to the practitioners.

3

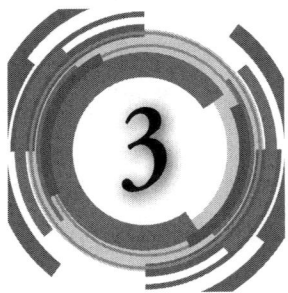

Temporary Privileges for Patient Care Needs

Anne Roberts, CPCS, CPMSM

CASE STUDY

Influenza season is here, and there is an influx of patients arriving in the emergency department (ED). There are not enough practitioners in the ED to handle the increased volume, and the hospital has decided to open an alternate care site for the low-acuity patients to be triaged. The alternate care site will be staffed with general practitioners and advanced practice professionals (APP), including physician assistants (PA) and nurse practitioners (NP). The hospital needs to determine what types of privileges are appropriate for those who are taking shifts in the alternate care site. Additionally, the medical staff services department, in collaboration with the APP and the supervising physician, must outline the supervision requirements as well as requirements for prescriptive authority (if required by the state board). The organization clearly has an immediate patient care need that must be addressed. What are the appropriate steps to take to meet this need?

What Qualifies as 'Immediate Patient Care Need'?

There are some circumstances when the granting of temporary privileges is essential in order for the organization to meet urgent or immediate patient care needs. Organizations should have policies that clearly outline their pre-established criteria for granting temporary privileges. Although expediting the process is important, medical services professionals (MSP) must ensure that each practitioner's current clinical competence is verified to protect patient safety and avoid potential negligent credentialing claims.

The following are some examples of situations that justify granting temporary privileges for an urgent or immediate patient care need:

- **Staffing issues:** A specialist takes an unexpected leave of absence, and there isn't a qualified practitioner to cover his or her patients; the medical staff may need to temporarily privilege another specialist to cover patients for the specialist on leave. Or, per the case study described above, there are not enough practitioners to care for the volume of patients, and the medical staff must grant practitioners temporary privileges to meet the urgent or immediate patient care needs.

- **Necessary expertise:** A patient needs specific care, treatment, or services, and there are currently no practitioners on the medical staff that either hold the appropriate privileges, or have the necessary expertise to provide such care, treatment or services. Temporary privileges may be granted for a specific patient care need.

- **Disaster:** A disaster plan for the organization has been implemented, and there is not sufficient staff to manage the influx of patients affected by the disaster. The medical staff can grant temporary privileges in accordance with its disaster privileging policy.

Developing a Temporary-Privileges Policy

Medical staffs should keep several things in mind when developing a temporary-privilege policy, including the following:

- Typically, when organizations grant temporary privileges for an urgent patient care need, it is for a specific patient or to provide specific care, treatment or services for a limited amount of time. For Joint Commission–accredited organizations, temporary privileges granted to a practitioner to meet an urgent or immediate patient care need cannot exceed 120 days.

- Granting temporary privileges does not mean that the medical staff must also grant the practitioner medical staff membership. Although temporary privileges can and often are granted to practitioners from within the organization, they also often are granted to those who come from outside the organization. In these cases, it is not necessary to grant them medical staff membership.

- The termination of temporary privileges typically does not afford a practitioner the right to due process.

When granting temporary privileges, at minimum organizations should verify that the practitioner holds a current, unrestricted state license and professional liability insurance that meets the minimum requirements set by the organization's governing board. To verify a practitioner's competence, the organization should ensure that:

- The individual meets the minimum threshold criteria outlined for the specialty in question, such as:

  - Board certification

  - Completion of a subspecialty residency or fellowship training program (typically these criteria can be easily verified by checking the practitioner's AMA profile)

- The anesthesiologist or practitioner who will be prescribing or administering narcotics has the appropriate state and federal narcotics licenses

- The practitioner is not on the Office of Inspector General's excluded parties list

- There are no National Practitioner Data Bank reports indicating prior competence or professional behavior concerns

Figure 3.1 is a temporary privileges request form that ensures the practitioner's information has been verified according to the organization's policies and procedures before granting temporary privileges. When time permits, MSPs should also attempt to obtain additional information as soon as possible. For example, if the privileges are going to be granted for a specified time period, the MSP should proceed by verifying other essential items typically required to privilege practitioners, such as a criminal background screening and a clinical evaluation from the practitioner's department chair at his or her primary admitting facility. Although temporary privileges may have been granted to meet an urgent or immediate patient care need, if information is discovered later during the credentialing process, the temporary privileges can be terminated for cause if needed, without due process, as long as this is clearly outlined in the organization's temporary-privilege policy.

FIGURE 3.1
TEMPORARY PRIVILEGES REQUEST FORM

To be completed by medical staff services:

Applicant Name: _____

Specialty/Division: _____

Effective Date of Temporary Privileges Desired: _____

1. Has the required information been verified according to policies and procedures? ____ Yes   ____ No

2. Have any red flags been identified in this file? If yes, please provide an explanation. ____ Yes (see attached) ____ No

3. Does this applicant meet the requirements as set forth in the policies and procedures? ____ Yes ____ No

Category 1 Temporary Privileges: Urgent Patient Care Need

❑ Applicant performs specialized procedure/services that no other practitioner on staff can perform (see attached details and recommendation from the applicable division chief).

❑ Patient volume exceeds the number of current physicians available in this subspecialty area. Applicant is needed to fulfill this patient care need (see attached request from the applicable division chief).

Category 2 Temporary Privileges:

❑ This applicant's credentials and privileges have been approved by the Credentials Committee and are awaiting review and approval from the Medical Executive Committee and the Board of Directors. There are no red flags that would preclude the applicant from qualifying for Category 2 temporary privileges.

_____   _____

Review and Approval - Director, Medical Staff Services   **Date**

        The Medical Staff's Guide to Overcoming Competence Assessment Challenges

---

FIGURE 3.1

TEMPORARY PRIVILEGES REQUEST FORM (CONT.)

Division Chief Approval:

I have reviewed the applicant's request for temporary privileges, along with the appropriate credentialing informa-tion, and make the following recommendation regarding the request for temporary privileges:

____ **Approve**   ____ **Deny**   ____ **Approve with conditions**

Comments: _____

_____

_____   _____

Signature, Division Chief   **Date**

NO	YES	REVIEWED/APPROVED BY:
❏	❏	President of the Medical/Dental Staff – **(TYPE NAME)** or designee (President-Elect or Credentials Chair) Signature: _____ Date: _____
❏	❏	**(TYPE NAME)**, Vice President of Medical Affairs as designee for **(TYPE NAME)**, Chief Executive Officer Signature: _____ Date: _____

As mentioned above, organizations should have a clear policy that outlines the criteria that they have developed for granting temporary privileges. The Joint Commission requires that accredited organizations outline the process in the medical staff bylaws, which should include the minimum criteria, a list of which practitioners can approve temporary privileges (include designees, if applicable), and the time frame in which they can be granted. The details of the process can be outlined in a separate policy or in the medical staff bylaws.

In the initial example regarding the influx of influenza patients that require additional staffing, the hospital would pool internal resources if available and grant temporary privileges to current practitioners if necessary to allow them to work in the temporary urgent care center. Temporary privileges for internal practitioners would only be required if the scope of practice in the urgent care center falls outside of their scope of privileges or if the clinic is located off-site. The hospital could also grant temporary privileges to external practitioners to fulfill this need.

Pendency of an Application/Committee Approval

The hospital can also grant temporary privileges if a complete, clean application (no significant red flags) has been reviewed and recommended without reservations by the appropriate department chair, and the application is just awaiting approval by the appropriate medical staff committees and governing body.

Your temporary-privilege policy should clearly outline what your organization considers red flags that would preclude an applicant from qualifying for temporary privileges and require full review and approval of his or her application by all applicable committees (e.g., credentials committee, medical executive committee [MEC], and the governing board). If your organization is Joint Commission–accredited, MS.06.01.11 outlines applications that should not be processed through an expedited approval process. Organizations typically use these same criteria as disqualifiers for temporary privileges.

Your credentialing policies should outline the time frame that the relevant committees and governing board must act on a completed application for temporary privileges. Additionally, some state statutes dictate the time frame in which the approval must occur. The organization should clearly define what is considered a complete application. When granting temporary privileges for an application that is pending committee approval, the duration of the temporary privileges should not exceed the time frame within which the committees are required to act on a completed application.

Temporary Privileges for Locum Tenens

Locum tenens physicians provide interim staffing, typically via contractual arrangements through a staffing firm. Hospitals, individual practitioners, and groups of practitioners often enter into agreements with staffing firms. The agreements outline whether the hospital will delegate the credentials verification function to the staffing firm or require credentials verification in-house. Often, when an organization contracts with a locum tenens firm, it is for an urgent staffing need that requires an expedited credentialing process. If the hospital has chosen to delegate the credentials verification function to the staffing agency, the processing time is reduced, as well as the frequency that the organization needs to grant temporary privileges.

If the hospital chooses to delegate the credentials verification function, the hospital is still responsible for ensuring that the practitioner meets the criteria required of other practitioners applying for clinical privileges, including demonstrated clinical competence for the privileges requested.

The verification information obtained by the staffing agency should be equivalent to that obtained by the medical staff services department. The medical staff should outline verification processes in the contract, and as well as a mechanism to audit the credentials verification practices of the staffing agency to ensure that they are meeting the credentialing expectations established by the hospital.

Although the staffing agency may have done the credentials verification, the credentials committee and MEC still need to make a recommendation, and the governing board is still responsible for the final decision.

The medical staff can reduce the incidence of temporary or locum tenens privileges by completing the routine credentialing verification processes and ensuring that medical staff leadership has sufficient time to review and recommend membership and/or privileges. In doing so, organizations reduce the risk of patient harm and legal challenges regarding the credentialing and privileging processes. Therefore, the medical staff services department should make every effort to reduce the use of locum tenens practitioners and reduce the use of temporary privileges being granted to locum tenens practitioners. Some recommended methods to accomplish this include:

- Remove language in medical staff governance documents that provides for locum tenens privileges. By doing so, the existing language outlining the routine processes for granting privileges would apply. Further, the current criteria regarding granting temporary privileges can also be applied to the candidate or the circumstances as appropriate.

- Identify and remedy circumstances that may require locum tenens coverage, (e.g., a single practitioner in a specialty).

- Encourage staff members to seek long-term coverage rather than episodic coverage.

- Request that the practitioner who will be providing the long-term coverage apply for privileges (without membership).

- Determine the staff member's reason for requesting coverage. If the coverage is isolated to the practitioner's office, then privileges are not needed in the acute care setting. Normal routine coverage arrangements can be applied.

- Create a preferred relationship with a locum tenens agency or agencies.

- Develop an agreement(s) to share appropriate credential verification information obtained by the agency, including all negative evaluations.

Most importantly, organizations should reduce the incidence of granting any privileges (temporary or locum tenens) without satisfying all components of the credentialing process using the following four steps:

- Step 1: Evaluate average turnaround time for processing applications

- Step 2: Compare to industry standard

- Step 3: Identify methods to streamline processes and reduce delays without compromising outcome

- Step 4: Ensure adequate resources for the credentialing and privileging functions

Reducing turnaround time can help reduce the need for temporary privileges in several ways, such as:

- If MSPs notify applicants, department chairs, and others in the organization of what the average turnaround time is, then they can better plan ahead and have an expectation of how long it will take. For example, if a department chair is recruiting candidates, and he knows that the average credentialing turnaround time is 60 to 90 days, he can keep that in mind when hiring new staff.

- Physicians who may not be employed by the organization but are submitting an application for membership and privileges can be told from the get-go to not expect privileges for at least 60 to 90 days (or whatever the average turnaround time is for the organization).

- Organizations that employ physicians should also take into consideration not only the amount of time it takes to credential someone for hospital privileges, but also how long it takes to get the physician enrolled in all of the health plans so that he or she can bill for services.

- The policy should outline justifiable reasons for granting temporary privileges, and these reasons should be communicated to the department chairs and those physician leaders who sign off/approve temporary privileges. Poor planning (such as someone out on vacation or not taking the average turnaround time into consideration when hiring someone) is not a justifiable reason for temporary privileges. Temporary privileges for patient care need are outlined earlier in the chapter.

Assessing the Competence of Proctors

Whenever an organization does not have a qualified specialist on staff, such as whenever a new procedure or technique is introduced to the organization, it may be necessary for the medical staff to grant temporary privileges to an external proctor to provide the necessary training and/or to monitor competence.

The medical staff should grant proctors from outside of the organization specific privileges for the area in which their expertise is needed, and the medical staff services department should verify their current clinical competence. Processing privileges for an external proctor is similar to granting temporary privileges, as they are typically not granted medical staff membership, they are not afforded the right to due process, and their privileges are granted for a specified amount of time. The proctors' privileges also typically include a statement that indicates whether they will intervene in the care of the patient or assume full care of the patient if it is clear that the physician being proctored is in need of assistance or there is any potential risk to the patient.

The minimum criteria for credentialing and verifying current clinical competence for proctors are typically the same as the criteria for granting temporary privileges; however, often additional competence verification requirements are needed.

For example, if the proctor is on-site to train physicians on the Da Vinci robot, the organization should verify that he or she has the necessary training and expertise from the vendor and other sources demonstrating specific training and competencies performing the procedures with the equipment.

Visiting Professors

Often, the university that a teaching hospital is affiliated with will allow visiting professors to work at their institution. The teaching hospital must have policies and procedures in place to outline the credentialing process for visiting professors if, as a part of their affiliation with the medical school, they will also be providing patient care services at the hospital. Most state medical licensing boards have specific requirements regarding visiting professors and have stipulations that any care they provide to patients is under the auspices of their affiliation with the medical school. Most organizations will either grant visiting professors time-limited temporary privileges or fully credential them, depending on how long they will be working at the university in the capacity of a visiting professor.

Hospitals that grant privileges to visiting professors need to ensure that the visiting professors meet the minimum threshold criteria for privileges. They must also clearly outline any restrictions that may be required to limit their practice to meet the guidelines required for visiting professors; for example, a practitioner's license is tied solely to his or her affiliation with the medical school, and therefore all activities are limited to that role. Often, privileges are granted for a period equivalent to the time frame that the state board has authorized.

4

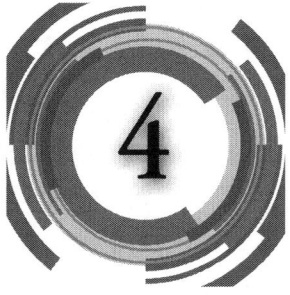

Attribution Challenges

Anne Roberts, CPCS, CPMSM

CASE STUDY

Mary, a medical staff quality coordinator, has been charged with gathering activity information for all practitioners for ongoing professional practice evaluations (OPPE). Some of the data that the medical staff has identified as being meaningful to review include:

- Number of admissions

- Average length of stay

- Number of procedures performed in both the inpatient and outpatient settings

- Number of consults responded to and average response time

- Number of patient referrals

Additionally, Mary has a list of OPPE indicators for each division that includes the need for denominator data (total common factors used for comparative data purposes). For example, for neurosurgery, denominator data may include the total number of shunts placed and the numerator would be the total shunt infections per surgeon. Other common examples of OPPE indicators are readmission rates, or, more specifically, readmission rates for congestive heart failure patients; length of stay or length of stay in ICU; drug utilization data; returns to surgery; and rate of normal pathology findings in patients undergoing hysterectomy. Mary is also charged with gathering other performance measures, such as total number of times a pharmacist was required to intervene for medication errors per practitioner and compliance with medical record documentation rules.

Mary requests the data from several departments, including admitting, information systems, medical records, pharmacy, and financial services. She quickly realizes when comparing the data submitted from each of the departments that there is a discrepancy. She presents the data to the medical staff leaders, and they identify that there must be errors in the way data are being attributed to practitioners. They now face the challenge of identifying at which step in the process the data are inaccurately attributed.

Patient Handoffs

One of the most common situations that causes attribution difficulties is when care of a patient is handed off to multiple practitioners. Often, staff will list in the medical record the name of the physician who admitted the patient; however throughout the patient's stay, the record is not updated when the care of the patient is handed off to other providers.

The practitioner primarily responsible for the care of the patient is typically referred to as the attending physician or attending practitioner, and this may change frequently, sometimes as often as after each shift. This is further clarified throughout this chapter.

Another attribution error can occur when the patient is admitted to one service and transferred to another service, yet the name of the attending physician is still listed as the admitting physician. This causes all data related to that patient to be attributed to the admitting physician instead of the attending physician, who has now assumed responsibility for the care of the patient.

The first step to ensuring accurate attribution is to define the roles of the practitioners. For example:

- **Admitting physician:** The medical staff member who has accepted and written orders for the patient to be admitted to the hospital.

- **Attending:** The physician who has the primary responsibility for directing the overall care of the patient. For example, on medical services, such as in an ICU or a hospitalist service, the physician who is accepting the primary responsibility for the care of the patient on any given day or shift is the attending physician of record. For procedures, the primary surgeon or proceduralist performing the procedure is the attending.

- **Consulting practitioner:** Whenever a consult is requested, the practitioner who is assigned to respond to the consult, sees the patient, and provides consultative recommendations (which may include transferring care of the patient to another service) is the consulting practitioner.

- **Primary care physician:** The physician with an established relationship with the patient (outside of the hospital) who provides general routine care or treatment for the patient.

- **Referring physician:** The physician who refers the patient to a specialist or to a hospital for admission to a teaching or hospitalist service or for evaluation at the emergency department.

- **Responsible practitioner:** Some hospitals do not allow advanced practice professionals (APP) to be members of the medical staff but will grant them privileges to provide a medical level of care in accordance with state law and organizational policies. Thus, the organization may use other terms to identify these practitioners, such as the responsible practitioner, rather than the attending. Additionally, in a teaching hospital, as residents or fellows are not considered attendings, this term may be used for them as well as for APPs.

Joe is a 49-year-old male who has arrived at the emergency department (ED) with severe chest pains. Joe was transported via ambulance from his general cardiologist's office. His cardiologist referred him directly to the ED due to the sudden onset of his symptoms and severity of his chest pain. The hospital staff lists the cardiologist as the referring physician, which allows the cardiologist to receive updates regarding the treatment that Joe receives while he is at the hospital so that he can better manage any subsequent care postdischarge.

When Joe arrives in the ED, the emergency physician quickly performs a history and physical, stabilizes the patient, and orders the appropriate tests, including an echocardiogram. He calls an interventional cardiologist for a consult to determine whether the patient needs to be taken to the cardiac catheterization lab immediately for a procedure to resolve any potential blockage. The consulting interventional cardiologist recommends that the patient be transferred to the catheterization lab for an interventional procedure. The medical record reflects that the interventional cardiologist is the consulting physician.

When the patient is transferred to the catheterization lab for the interventional procedure, the interventional cardiologist who is scheduled to perform the procedure is documented as the attending physician of record for that procedure. Due to complications in the catheterization lab, the patient requires immediate transfer to the operating room for open-heart surgery by a cardiovascular and thoracic surgeon. When the surgeon assumes the care of the patient, he is listed as the attending of record for the heart surgery.

After surgery, the surgeon makes arrangements for Joe to be admitted to the cardiac ICU for postoperative care. The surgeon is listed as the admitting physician and remains listed as the attending of record until such time that he or she hands the care of the patient off to an ICU attending physician. Once in the cardiac ICU, the care of the patient is now in the hands of an ICU attending, who shares service or call responsibilities with other ICU attendings. Depending on how the organization sets its call schedules, the ICU attending may change at every shift or after a specified block of time (for example, the attending may be on service for a few days or a couple of weeks). The medical record reflects the transition each time the attending hands the care of the patient off to the next attending.

Once you have defined the roles within your organization, it is then important to identify when and how care is transferred to other members of the care team and how this should be documented appropriately in the medical record. Below is an example of a patient's hospital stay and how each of these physicians interact with the patient.

As you can see from this example, patient care can change hands multiple times throughout a hospital stay. It is important to ensure that each time the care is transitioned, the responsible attending of record is appropriately documented, not only for billing purposes, but also to accurately track and attribute quality data related to the patient and volume/activity data for each practitioner.

In the example given above, it is important to ensure that the emergency physician is accurately attributed to the patient in case there is ever a question related to the care provided in the ED. It is also important to attribute this patient encounter to the appropriate attending for billing and activity tracking (e.g., reviewing the volume of patients seen by this attending during an OPPE cycle or identifying how many patients presenting to the ED with cardiac arrest have been treated by this physician, etc.).

The interventional cardiologist who responded to the consult request in the ED also needs to be appropriately attributed to the patient for similar reasons. There may be a question or concern related to the evaluation and subsequent recommendations that he or she provided after seeing the patient. In addition, the organization needs to collect data for billing and trending activity for the physician (e.g., how many consults did the physician respond to and did he or she respond to the consult in a timely manner?).

The cardiologist who performed the interventional procedure in the catheterization lab may not necessarily be the same cardiologist who responded to the consult in the ED. Attributing the procedure to the physician who performed the procedure is important for billing and activity data and to ensure that any complications that may have occurred are tracked and trended for quality purposes. If there was indeed a complication, the organization should make certain that it is attributed to the right attending to ensure appropriate performance monitoring. The same applies to the cardiovascular and thoracic surgeon who performed the open-heart surgery.

When the patient is admitted to the ICU, ensuring that the change of attending is appropriately documented is important not only for quality, billing, and activity tracking purposes, but also to ensure that should an issue arise, the staff in the ICU can quickly identify which attending should be called.

The multi-specialty management of Joe's chest pain is a common occurrence for the majority of patients who are admitted to acute care facilities. Thus, the importance of accurately documenting the roles and responsibilities of each practitioner providing care becomes vital for accurate attribution of the care provided by each individual practitioner. The patient's clinical record is the primary source for this information.

Teaching Service

At teaching hospitals, several other layers of practitioners are involved in the care of the patient, including medical students, residents, fellows, and allied health students. Many students are allowed to document in the medical record; however, their notes are viewed as information only for teaching purposes. Residents and fellows, as they progress through their training, are granted permission to provide patient care under specified levels of supervision. Ensuring accurate attribution of patient care to the appropriate resident and/or fellow is just as important as other members of the care team. In almost all cases, an attending cannot bill for care provided by a resident unless certain supervision requirements are met. For quality of care purposes, attributing medical decision-making to the appropriate practitioner is always important. In addition to accurate practitioner attribution, teaching hospitals must also review and analyze whether the care was provided under the appropriate level of supervision.

Medical staff rules and regulations generally outline the responsibilities of supervising physicians as they relate to medical record documentation. For example, a physician may be required to provide a countersignature or review and affirm a plan of care suggested by a trainee or APP prior to the care being delivered.

Advanced Practice Professionals

Attribution of patient care for APPs has the same implications as it does for physicians in regard to monitoring quality data and billing. Most APPs are allowed to bill independently for their services; therefore, they must be able to appropriately track the care that they provide to ensure accurate billing.

Many organizations continue to struggle with appropriately attributing care provided by APPs, in particular, when there are specific supervision requirements in place that must be met before the patient encounter can be closed. When this occurs, coding these encounters appropriately for billing purposes can be a significant challenge. This is generally due to limited resources and/or technological capabilities. Organizations must find a way to resolve these challenges for many reasons, including patient safety, performance improvement endeavors, risk management, and regulatory and accreditation requirements. Until organizations are capable of accurately capturing the activity of APPs, a temporary solution is to request that APPs provide a log of patients seen. This may be created manually by the APP or may be produced by generating a copy of the APP's billing records.

Another option to ensure appropriate attribution for APPs is to attribute the outcome data to both the physician and the APP, as appropriate. For example, attribution of a post-operative infection would be to both the surgeon and the assisting PA, unless the record documents a clear break of technique or complication caused by one of the individuals. Similarly, a readmission for congestive heart failure would be attributed to both the internist and the NP who cared for the patient while in the hospital. Lastly, the lengthy hospital course for an uneventful vaginal delivery would be attributed to the obstetrician as well as the midwife who cared for the patient.

Additionally, whenever a case has been evaluated by a peer review committee and it is determined that the care provided deviated from expected standards, the committee should attribute the case separately to each member of the care team as appropriate. For example, the committee would need to identify whether specific concerns regarding the care, treatment or services that did not meet expectations should be attributed to the APP (or other members of the care team) rather than solely to the attending physician.

Another reason to accurately attribute care provided by APPs is similar to the circumstances of a resident or fellow. In most states, even if an APP is allowed to bill for certain services, physicians are still required to supervise. The organization should not only be ensuring that patient care is attributed to the correct APP for billing and quality purposes, but it should also be monitoring whether the appropriate supervision (as required by the state board and/or organization's policy) is being provided.

Therefore, when a complication is identified and attributed to the APP, it is also important to determine if the complication resulted from the lack of appropriate supervision. If so, then the complication and supervision concerns would also be attributed to the responsible attending.

Attribution Issues and Solutions

In the case study at the beginning of the chapter, if Mary and the medical staff leaders tackle the attribution challenges outlined throughout this chapter, they will be able to improve the denominator data used for each department's OPPE indicators, improve the accuracy of all performance measures, and provide more accurate practitioner data (or group data) as needed throughout the organization to enable the organization to effectively measure performance.

There are times when it becomes logistically difficult (if not impossible) to attribute an outcome measure to a particular practitioner. In the case study presented at the beginning of this chapter, Joe was admitted with chest pain. Let's say that his overall length of stay was three days longer than the average. Three days of this added stay was while Joe was in the ICU. Further, while Joe was in the ICU, four intensivists cared for him.

The organization needs to ask the question, "Can we accurately attribute the additional length of stay to one practitioner?" The answer will generally be, "Probably not." In this situation, many organizations have chosen to attribute this length of stay to all four intensivists (or to the entire group of practitioners—physicians and APPs). Thus, the group is asked to review the patient's care and justify the need for the additional stay in the ICU.

This solution is not uncommon and can be applied to large and small partnerships and group practices. Patients often see multiple practitioners within a partnership or group depending on availability. The patient may not receive the majority of his or her care from the physician who is considered the primary care provider or specialist. Additionally, multiple physicians often take call for each other's patients.

Given these practice pattern realities, it is logical and reasonable to attribute the care to the partnership and/or group. If a deviation from the norm is noted, the practitioners involved are asked to collectively review and comment on the data. Another way to evaluate management of a patient population is to assess the outcome by targeting a particular diagnosis—such as chest pain (such as in the example earlier in the chapter). Thus, the outcome is attributed to the appropriate practitioners involved in the care.

To accurately assess practice patterns attributed to more than one practitioner, MSPs should ensure that they maintain an accurate list of practitioner partnerships and groups. Examples of multi-physician practice pattern data that can be used for various purposes by the hospital include, but are not limited to, volume data (such as referrals or admissions), clinical management and outcomes data, and billing/revenue data for each group as a whole.

Most credentialing databases are set up to easily attribute physicians to a partnership or group practice by their group name or tax ID number.

5

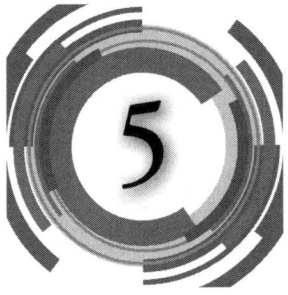

Ongoing Competence Challenges and Validation at Reappointment

Anne Roberts, CPCS, CPMSM

CASE STUDY

While reviewing Dr. Smith's ongoing professional practice evaluation (OPPE) data for the past six months, his department chair notices that Dr. Smith's average patient length of stay is longer than that of anyone else in the department. The chair has several questions and concerns that he must resolve before he can make an informed decision regarding how to address what appears to be a potential quality concern. According to the data provided, Dr. Smith appears to be a significant outlier from his peers in this regard; the question is why. The medical staff services department is called in to assist the department chair in obtaining the answers to his questions so that he can make the appropriate recommendations.

After Initial Appointment, What Are the Next Steps in Assessing Competence?

As outlined in Chapter 1, once the medical staff and governing board grant a practitioner clinical privileges (either at the time of initial appointment or at the time that the practitioner has been granted new or additional privileges), the practitioner should undergo an initial focused professional practice evaluation (FPPE) to confirm his or her competence. If the practitioner does not currently have sufficient evidence of current clinical competence, and your organization has decided to allow him or her to obtain that competence through onsite education and training, the practitioner can undergo supervised precepting, as outlined in Chapter 7.

Once the practitioner successfully completes his or her initial FPPE, the medical staff is then responsible for ensuring that the practitioner maintains current clinical competence for all privileges granted, monitoring the quality of care provided by the practitioner, and reviewing and monitoring the practitioner's overall performance. To monitor competence on an ongoing basis, organizations must develop systems to collect and assess performance data to measure the quality of care their practitioners deliver and ensure that the organization permits practitioners to maintain only those privileges they are competent to perform.

Often, negligent credentialing claims are based on allegations that the organization failed to ensure that a practitioner was competent to provide specified care, treatment, or services. Organizations should ensure that they have done their due diligence to not only verify initial competence but to also establish a comprehensive process to monitor and review practitioners' ongoing competence.

Monitoring a practitioner's overall performance is a comprehensive, data-driven process. Most organizations collate these data into a central department for tracking and trending and/or use commercially available databases to help streamline the process. Performance data that should be monitored on an ongoing basis include but are not limited to the following:

- Department-specific quality metrics (see the OPPE section later in this chapter)

- Quality metrics identified by the organization that can be tracked and measured for each practitioner (e.g., average length of patient stay as noted in the example above, unplanned returns to the emergency department or ICU, timely patient discharge, etc.)

- Compliance with medical record documentation requirements (e.g., countersignatures; appropriate documentation of verbal orders; thorough, accurate, and timely documentation; etc.)

- Medication reconciliation compliance (e.g., review any discrepancies noted by the pharmacy or error rates attributed to the practitioner)

- Complaints or grievances reported from patients/families

- Performance concerns documented by the department chair (e.g., collegiality, meeting attendance, feedback from medical students/residents, etc.)

- Peer review data (e.g., clinical or behavioral concerns, policy or compliance violations, etc.)

- Maintenance of current credentials (e.g., number of times practitioner allowed license, Drug Enforcement Administration, insurance, or other credentials to expire, resulting in automatic suspension)

- Ongoing monitoring of state medical board investigations/sanctions, National Practitioner Data Bank (NPDB) updates, and Office of Inspector General (OIG) queries to ensure the practitioner is not on the excluded parties list

- Complaints or concerns reported from employees, the compliance department, or peers

- Overall compliance with hospital policies, code of conduct, medical staff bylaws, and rules and regulations

- Data from patient/family satisfaction surveys

- Any other data identified by the organization as being meaningful and measurable performance data

Pulling these data together can be challenging and is an organization-wide effort. Please see Chapter 4 for more details on how to ensure that the data being collected are appropriately attributed to the right practitioner to help improve the integrity of the data being reviewed and ensure meaningful evaluations.

Developing Indicators for Ongoing Competence Assessment

An important step in developing an effective OPPE process is to identify the types of data that will provide meaningful information about a practitioner's performance and develop systems to collect that data. Hospitals generally gather data related to patient care and measure the outcomes (good and bad) based on several factors. The specific quality indicators chosen to measure competence will vary by organization. The type of services that the facility offers, organizational culture, and patient volume all affect which indicators the organization chooses. One of the first steps toward choosing meaningful indicators is to answer the following questions:

- What data does your organization wish to track?

- Are the data relevant and meaningful?

- Is there a mechanism to gather the data and ensure accuracy?

When evaluating indicators, the medical staff should identify whether the information is relevant and meaningful to the practitioner's performance. Will gathering this data provide meaningful information that can be used to truly measure practitioner performance? Additionally, indicators should be reviewed on an as-needed basis to determine whether they continue to be meaningful.

Additionally, organizations need to take into consideration whether the data are currently available and, if they aren't, what steps the organization must take to gather and collect the data for each indicator identified.

For example, some indicator data will be available only at the department level and will require chart audits to pull the data; documentation requirements are tracked by the medical records department; infection rates are typically tracked by the infection control department; and medication errors are tracked by the pharmacy. If the medical staff determines that the requested data are meaningful but are not currently available, the organization would need to work collaboratively with the applicable parties within the organization to develop a tracking process for the data.

When developing quality indicators, physician leaders should take the following into consideration:

- **Attribution:** Can the indicator measure individual physician performance with reasonable reliability and accuracy?

- **Availability:** Can you get the data today, or will it take time to collect? Is there currently a data source available with the needed information, or will a process to collect the data need to be developed?

- **Benefit:** Is the cost to measure the data worth the potential improvement should the indicator be implemented?

Implementing OPPE and Addressing Competence Concerns

Once the organization structures its OPPE process to collect data and establishes meaningful quality indicators, the next steps are to:

- Collect and collate the data

- Communicate the results to applicable parties as determined by the organization

- Take necessary action to address any concerns

Although the task of generating an individual practitioner profile report can seem daunting, once these reports are fine-tuned and the integrity of the data is confirmed, they become an essential tool for monitoring practitioners' competence. As discussed earlier in this chapter, the documentation the organization maintains regarding ongoing competence reviews should be comprehensive, as it may be used later should a claim of negligent credentialing arise or should action need to be taken against a practitioner whose performance has been identified as falling below the expected standard.

Once the profiles are generated, the medical staff determines who should review and assess the data. Often, organizations will only report the data to the department chairs and leave the chair to communicate results to the individual practitioners. Once the attribution challenges outlined in Chapter 4 are addressed, and there is a comfort level in the integrity of the data, organizations may decide to provide direct feedback to each individual practitioner.

Some organizations have chosen to have all OPPE data reported up through a medical staff committee (performance improvement, peer review, or credentials committee) to provide a higher level of oversight and accountability to ensure department chairs are addressing concerns in a timely, consistent, and meaningful manner.

Addressing Competence Concerns Identified During the Ongoing Review Process

During OPPE, if a practitioner has not met the expected and established performance measures, the department chair and/or appropriate committee should clearly document how the concern was addressed. In the example at the beginning of this chapter, during an OPPE review, the department chair noted that Dr. Smith's average patient length of stay is longer than that of his peers. To evaluate why this is the case, the chair needs to take the following into consideration:

- **Volume data:** How many patients does Dr. Smith see in comparison to his peers? The chair notes that Dr. Smith sees 25% more patients than anyone else in the department.

- **Diagnosis/disposition:** To truly compare length of stay, the chair must look at the types of patients that Dr. Smith has admitted in comparison to his peers. He notes that the patients whose lengths of stay were longer for Dr. Smith had the same diagnosis/disposition as several of his peers' patients; therefore, he was not treating higher-acuity patients than his peers.

- **Timely discharge:** The next thing the department chair evaluated was the time Dr. Smith wrote discharge orders for each of the patients whose lengths of stay were longer than those of his peers. He found that while most of the practitioners in the department were writing discharge orders prior to 10 a.m. the day of discharge, Dr. Smith's discharge orders were often not written until noon.

Based on the information given above, the chair determined that the reason Dr. Smiths' average patient length of stay was longer than that of his peers was because he was seeing more patients and not writing his discharge orders in a timely manner. To address these concerns, the chair met with Dr. Smith to review the data and identify what could be done to help Dr. Smith write his discharge orders in a more timely manner.

For example, the department chair can suggest that Dr. Smith identify patients who are ready for discharge the evening before and, if appropriate, write the order for discharge at that time rather than waiting until the morning or day of discharge. By doing so, it allows the staff to proactively prepare the patient for discharge and expedites the discharge process first thing in the morning, so long as there were not any changes overnight to the patient's condition that would warrant re-evaluation by the attending physician.

Whenever a performance concern, outlier, or red flag is noted during the OPPE process, the department chair should make a notation regarding what, if any, action the organization needs to take. For example, Dr. Smith's department chair documented his findings as to why Dr. Smith's average patient length of stay was longer than that of his peers and what steps were put into place to address this concern. Even if that action is simply to continue monitoring and reassess during the next OPPE data review, this action should be clearly documented in the practitioner's OPPE profile.

For additional information on developing quality indicators and implementing a step-by- step systematic approach to OPPE, please see *The Complete Guide to OPPE*, published by HCPro, Inc., available at *www.hcmarketplace.com*.

FPPE for Cause

Although FPPE is assigned for all new privileges, it can also be assigned to a practitioner for cause, meaning something specific triggered a review of the practitioner's performance. OPPE is a continuous, ongoing review of a practitioner's performance, but if concerns are identified through OPPE, the department chair may assign FPPE to address the concerns and monitor improvement. When performance issues are identified, the steps the medical staff should take to resolve the performance issues must be clearly defined. This means that the FPPE plan should be customized for the practitioner in question and must clearly outline the requirements, such as:

- Education: specific educational opportunities related to the concern identified

- Precepting: identify if precepting is appropriate and available

- Proctoring: identify if proctoring is appropriate to address the concern

- Who is accountable for monitoring the progress plan

- How the improvement will be measured and documented

     The Medical Staff's Guide to Overcoming Competence Assessment Challenges

FPPE plans implemented for cause must be conducted in a timely manner to ensure patients receive safe, quality care from competent practitioners. The Joint Commission standards indicate that the decision to assign a period of performance monitoring to further assess current competence is based on the evaluation of a practitioner's current clinical competence, practice behavior, and ability to perform the requested privilege(s). When a concern is identified with a specific procedure or specific treatment plan, the other privileges held by the practitioner should not be affected.

If a practitioner takes a leave of absence (LOA), particularly a medical LOA, depending on the length of the LOA and circumstances, the medical staff may choose to require the individual to undergo FPPE when he or she returns to practice. The FPPE is customized for the individual based on the situation and could include proctoring, documentation of continuing medical education credits earned during the absence, etc. For example, if a practitioner has been out on leave for more than six months, the FPPE would be customized at the discretion of the department chair and the credentials committee. They would need to identify any specific concerns that should be addressed to ensure that, although the practitioner was out of practice for six months, he or she has maintained current clinical competence. Also, if there were health concerns, the department chair and credentials committee should discuss how to best implement a customized FPPE plan to ensure the practitioner's ability to provide safe, quality care has not been affected by those health concerns.

Competence Assessment at Reappointment

At the time of reappointment for medical staff members or advanced practice professionals (APP), the department chair should review all OPPE data from the past two years. This not only reminds the chair of any performance issues that have been addressed through the normal OPPE process, but he or she can also see whether anything has changed since the last appointment or whether there are any positive or negative trends that have developed in the past 24 months.

In addition to reporting internal OPPE data, the medical staff services department confirms that the practitioner has maintained current licensure and certification, reviews data from the NPDB, ensures that the practitioner has not been added to the OIG's excluded practitioners list, and runs another criminal background check.

Obtaining a clinical evaluation from the department chair at the practitioner's primary admitting facility is also important at the time of reappointment to document current clinical competence. The medical staff services department should also obtain case logs from the primary organization—internally obtained if yours is the primary location of practice, and externally obtained if the majority of the individual's practice is elsewhere.

It is important to not only obtain volume information but quality outcome data if possible. For APPs, clinical evaluations should be obtained from the supervising physician(s) if applicable or from the department chair in the area where he or she has been granted clinical privileges. The medical staff services department should obtain peer references if the above data are not available, if there is insufficient peer review data available, or there is a not a member of the staff in the same clinical discipline who can evaluate the practitioner. If the low-volume practitioner participates in teaching, confidential resident or medical student evaluation data can also be obtained for review.

Confirming a practitioner's health status at reappointment is also a requirement. Health status can be confirmed by obtaining an attestation from the applicant, verifying through clinical evaluations or peer reference, or if necessary, a physical exam and release from the practitioner's primary care practitioner.

Allied Health Annual Competence Reviews

Unlike APPs and medical staff members, competence evaluations for allied health professionals (AHP) is not onerous. For Joint Commission–accredited organizations, the HR standards require that AHPs have the same education, training, and competence requirements as their employed equivalents. For example, if the hospital employs surgical technicians/assistants and it allows medical staff members to bring their own surgical technicians/assistants in to assist them in the operating room, the credentialed surgical technicians/assistants and the employed surgical technicians/assistants have equivalent requirements. Typically, medical staff services departments will collaborate with the HR department to align job descriptions and competence requirements. If there is not an employed equivalent to a credentialed AHP, then the hospital is responsible for creating an appropriate description of the individual's responsibilities and required qualifications. The HR department would typically involve the requesting physician, pertinent medical staff leaders (such as the department chair or section chief), the credentials committee, and/or an AHP committee (if one exists).

Note: The Centers for Medicare & Medicaid Services require privileging for registered nurse first assistants, surgical assistants, etc., who perform surgical procedures. Included in the definition of surgical procedures are suturing, closing, manipulation of tissue, etc. Thus, regardless of who employs the RNFA or surgical assistant (hospital or physician) CMS requires these individuals be privileged if they are performing these functions. The Joint Commission standards do not include this requirement.

The Joint Commission also requires that the competence evaluation for an AHP is equivalent to that of an employed equivalent. Most organizations review their employees' performance on an annual basis; therefore, AHP evaluations should align with what the organization does for its employees.

For the competence evaluation of AHPs, at a minimum, organizations should ensure that the AHP and his or her sponsoring physician(s) review the position/job description annually to ensure that there have been no changes. The medical staff services department should also obtain a clinical evaluation from the sponsoring physician. Feedback can also be obtained from administrative supervisors for the area in which the AHP is providing services; for example, for a dental assistant who accompanies a dentist to the operating room, the nurse supervisor for the operating room can likely attest to whether the dental assistant complies with operating room policies and procedures, such as sterile technique, and whether he or she works collegially with other staff.

Ongoing competence evaluation is a comprehensive process. When done well, the data can be used for continuous performance improvement initiatives and help to ensure that practitioners are providing safe, quality patient care.

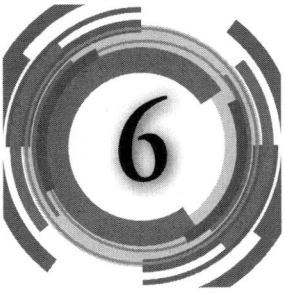

6 Assessing the Competence of APPs

Frances M. Ponsioen, CPMSM, CPCS

The director of medical staff services at Best Hospital in Town recognized that the current process for credentialing advanced practice professionals (APP) needed to change so that the facility was in compliance with various regulatory standards. The director identified the types of practitioners that were approved by the board of trustees to provide services within the facility and has been working diligently with medical staff leadership to make the necessary changes to the credentialing and privileging process for all APPs.

The director worked with a team that consisted of a representative from the HR department, a representative from nursing education, and a credentialing specialist from the medical staff services department. First, they identified the types of practitioners that needed to be pulled from the current allied health professionals (AHP) category, such as registered nurse (RN), licensed vocational nurse, and surgical scrub technician, because they are not providing a medical level of care and therefore are not required to go through the more rigorous privileging process.

Second, the team developed a process to transition this group of allied health staff (sometimes referred to as clinical assistants [CA]) over to a process more in line with HR and the requirements established for employees. Together, the medical staff services department and HR worked to identify the differences in education and certification, with the goal of aligning a standard set of qualifications for the employed RN and a nonemployed RN, as well as other CA.

Once there was a clear separation between CAs and APPs and a process had been developed and assumed by HR, the medical staff director was faced with addressing the evaluation and assessment of the APPs. What should she do?

The Center for Medicare & Medicaid Services (CMS)'s *Conditions of Participation* (*CoP*) provide for the governing body to have the authority, in accordance with state law and scope of practice, to appoint and/or grant privileges to some types of non-physician practitioners, such as:

- Physician assistant (PA)

- Nurse practitioner (NP)

- Clinical nurse specialist

- Certified registered nurse anesthetist (CRNA)

- Certified nurse-midwife

- Clinical social worker

- Clinical psychologist

- Registered dietitian or nutrition professional

Additionally, the CMS *CoP* surgical services §482.51(a)(4), state that hospitals must specify surgical privileges for each practitioner who performs surgical tasks. The *CoP*s state:

> "…if the hospital utilizes RNFAs [registered nurse first assistant], surgical PAs, or other non MD/DO surgical assistants, then the organization must establish qualifications, criteria, and a credentialing process to grant specific privileges … Important surgical tasks include: opening and closing, dissecting tissue, removing tissue, harvesting grafts, transplanting tissue, administering anesthesia, implanting devices and placing invasive lines."

The Interpretive Guidelines state that the hospital must specify the surgical privileges for each practitioner who performs surgical tasks, including RNFAs, NPs, surgical PAs, and surgical technicians. Hospitals that use RNFAs, surgical PAs, or other non-MD/DO surgical assistants must develop the following:

> "…criteria, qualifications and a credentialing process to grant specific privileges to individual practitioners based on each individual practitioner's compliance with the privileging/credentialing criteria and in accordance with Federal and State laws and regulations. This would include surgical services tasks conducted by these practitioners while under the supervision of an MD/DO."

The Joint Commission standards also require that PAs and advanced practice registered nurses (APRN) be privileged through a medical staff process. Standards that previously provided for PAs and APRNs to be processed through an equivalent process were disallowed in late 2010/early 2011 for hospitals that are utilizing The Joint Commission to achieve deemed status for Medicare/Medicaid participation.

In essence, every organization seeking deemed status is accountable to the CMS requirement for those individuals providing a "medical level of care" to be privileged. This requirement aligns with additional requirements for establishing competence for requested privileges (e.g., focused professional practice evaluation [FPPE], ongoing professional practice evaluation [OPPE], period appraisal, performance monitoring).

All Joint Commission Medical Staff standards are applicable, including recommendation by the organized medical staff and approval by the governing body. APPs who provide medical level of care include:

- PA

- APRN

  - NPs

  - Certified nurse midwives

  - CRNAs

  - Clinical nurse specialists

Collecting Data on APP Performance

Unless your medical staff services department adopted the "equivalent process" for verifying the education, training, licensure, and competence of AHPs (like the process for all privileged medical staff members) previously provided for in The Joint Commission standards, credentialing and privileging an APP has not been a recent challenge or a change for most medical staff services departments. Although no longer allowed for Joint Commission organizations seeking deemed status, the equivalent process was approved by the governing body and included:

- Documented evaluation of the applicant's credentials and the applicant's current competence

- Peer recommendations

- Input from individuals and committees, including the medical executive committee, to make an informed decision regarding requests for privileges

For most entities, unless they had a very large group of employed APPs, the equivalent process provided very little benefit. Therefore, the verification and maintenance of the APP was likely processed under the same guidelines and rules as physicians on the medical staff. In the case study at the beginning of the chapter, the challenge that the director and medical staff leadership face is bringing the assessment of the APP in line with the regulatory standards, which require APPs to undergo a similar form of performance measurement as physicians (e.g., FPPE and OPPE).

For those hospitals utilizing the equivalent process, The Joint Commission's clarification set the expectations that the APP is to be included in the FPPE and OPPE requirements under the medical staff process, not an "equivalent process." Although APRNs may practice independently in some organizations (if the organization and state law allow), the APP is traditionally viewed as a physician extender and does not practice within a hospital or healthcare system independently. APPs often practice under a collaborative or supervisory agreement with a qualified physician. However, APPs provide a medical level of care, which requires the facility to ensure that the APP is privileged and has the appropriate qualifications and competencies.

The competence assessment process varies among facilities. However, the process should be consistent for all licensed independent practitioners (LIP) and non-LIPs who are privileged under the medical staff. Unfortunately, the challenge in adhering to policy will be in the collection of the competence data for the APP, because in most cases the data are tied to the attending physician and not directly attributed to the APP. In addition, not all healthcare institutions are able to electronically capture activity or patient data for the APP if they are not the primary or attending practitioner.

Similar to the process that was used for developing the AHP evaluation process, the medical staff director in the case study at the beginning of the chapter will need to identify a number of experts, both internally and externally, who can assist with how the APP competence assessment process needs to be organized. Members from the quality department, medical records, and nursing administration will be key members of the team, and APPs should be part of the process. It will also be helpful if a few APPs are included. Understanding APPs' day-to-day experience within the organization will help the team create a process that works. Designating an APP committee to carry out FPPE and OPPE processes could improve the amount of data available for APP activity.

 The Medical Staff's Guide to Overcoming Competence Assessment Challenges

Prospective review, concurrent review (proctoring), or retrospective review are examples of the various ways to conduct a focused review or to evaluate privileged practitioners. The medical staff should work with APPs to define specific quality indicators and to collect data on an ongoing basis. Many APP disciplines may be evaluated utilizing the same quality indicators as their physician counterparts (e.g., CRNA and anesthesiologist; CNM and OB/GYN). If it is difficult or impossible to gather patient records showing that the APP participated in patient care, then the medical services professional (MSP) may reach out to the APP and request a list of patient records in which the APP was involved. For organizations that are still challenged with attributing care to the APP, it is helpful to both parties if the APP is notified ahead of time of the need to keep a list of activity for ongoing review. Once that list has been provided, a random number of records can be pulled and retrospectively reviewed by a peer or a physician, utilizing the same review forms that are used for physician review. However, it may be more appropriate to develop a review form that is tailored to the APP and the medical care that he or she provides under the supervision of or in collaboration with the sponsoring physician, including the documentation of consultation with the physician as appropriate.

When assessing competence of APPs, it is valuable to obtain an evaluation from the employing or supervising physician if applicable. MSPs should provide the individual with education regarding the form's purpose and content. An evaluation from a relevant hospital staff member who has routinely observed the practice of the APP should be obtained to make sure that the practitioner is adhering to hospital policies and procedures and codes of conduct. An operating room supervisor could provide an evaluation of a PA who has first assistant duties, as could an anesthesiologist.

Other methods to gather data include obtaining peer recommendations, evaluating patient and staff complaints, and reviewing incident reports involving APPs.

The medical staff also needs to determine a schedule for the APP evaluation that is manageable by both the medical staff services and quality departments. The evaluation schedule will vary depending on the organization, but it typically would mirror the time frame defined for other privileged practitioners. For Joint Commission–accredited facilities, it makes sense to have three periods of OPPE align with the 24-month reappointment cycle, resulting in OPPE reporting every eight months, or three times within the reappointment cycle. Conversely, a shorter reporting period (e.g., a six-month interval), goes beyond what The Joint Commission requires as "routine reporting" and utilizes additional scarce resources to perform the review. Other accrediting bodies (e.g., Healthcare Facilities Accreditation Program and Det Norske Veritas) are not as prescriptive, requiring periodic appraisal, monitoring, or collection of performance data.

Routinely providing APPs with performance reviews can help APPs improve their performance. Comparing data among practitioners will encourage practitioners to stop and question their own practices when they find that their performance is below par or average. Two targets resulting in three levels of performance will serve as a tool for improvement even if the practitioner is performing within the standard. Figure 6.1 depicts this concept.

FIGURE 6.1
PERFORMANCE TARGETS

Using targets to reduce bias and create an improvement culture

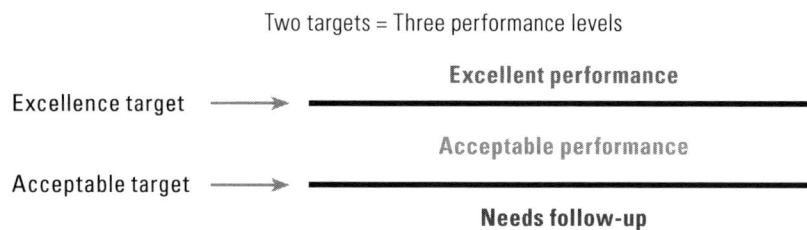

Two targets = Three performance levels

Excellent performance

Excellence target ⟶ ─────────────────────

Acceptable performance

Acceptable target ⟶ ─────────────────────

Needs follow-up

Cultural effect: Drives physician improvement

- Recognizes top performers

- Stimulates self-improvement of the middle

- Addresses potentially poor performance

As stated previously, developing a feedback report for the APP may be a bit different from the one issued to physicians due to the differences in their practices. However, some feedback reports, particularly for certified nurse midwives and OB/GYNs or CRNA and anesthesiologists, may look very similar.

We suggest that the medical staff services department send an evaluation form to the APP's sponsoring physician and/or a peer who can attest to the practitioner's ability to meet the Accreditation Council for Graduate Medical Education's and American Board of Medical Specialties' six core competencies:

 The Medical Staff's Guide to Overcoming Competence Assessment Challenges

- Patient care

- Medical/clinical knowledge

- Practice-based learning and improvement

- Interpersonal and communication skills

- Professionalism

- Systems-based practice

The evaluation form can be completed based on the peer's or physician's direct observation of the APP or as a tool that can be completed with a retrospective or concurrent chart review. Figure 6.2 is a sample APP evaluation form based on the six core competencies. The form can be sent to the APP's sponsoring physician and/or a peer who can attest to the practitioner's ability to meet the six core competencies. The form can be completed based on direct observation of the APP or retrospective or concurrent chart review.

Consider the following examples as specific measures within two of the competence areas:

- Interpersonal and communication skills: Does the APP work collaboratively with physicians and other healthcare professionals to provide patient-centered care?

- Interpersonal and communication skills: Does the APP accurately and adequately document and record information regarding the care process for medical, legal, quality, and financial purposes?

- Patient care: Can the APP perform medical and surgical procedures that are considered essential in the area of practice?

In the case of insufficient clinical activity, the medical staff may wish to send out a peer reference form to individuals who have been identified as a peer and/or associated with the APP, such as the supervising or sponsoring physician. The reference form should specifically address the requirements of the organization's accrediting body and can include the six core competencies in addition to questions related to individual observation and/or experience with the APP. The responses to the peer reference can then be reviewed by the appropriate reviewing body (e.g., department chair, credentials committee, and/or medical executive committee) in conjunction with any internal data or activity.

FIGURE 6.2

ALLIED HEALTH PROFESSIONAL COMPETENCY EVALUATION
ANP, APRN, CNS, CCP, FNP, Midwife, NP, NNP, PA, Psychologist

Applicant Name: _____   ID# _____

Sponsoring Physician: _____

Clinical Specialty: _____

Competency	Required Skill	Met	Not Met	Comment
			Evaluation	
Patient Care	Demonstrates caring and respectful behaviors when interacting with patients and families			
	Gathers essential and accurate patient information			
	Performs and dictates the H&P and discharge summary in a timely and accurate manner			
	Works collaboratively in a team atmosphere			
	Maintains clinical knowledge, skills and attitudes			
	Demonstrates proficient and appropriate use of procedural skills, both diagnostic and therapeutic			
	Adheres to medical staff policies and procedures			
Medical Knowledge	Demonstrates good investigatory and analytic thinking			
	Demonstrates knowledge and application of basic sciences			
Practice-Based Learning & Improvement	Analyzes own practice for needed improvements			
	Uses information communication and technology			

    The Medical Staff's Guide to Overcoming Competence Assessment Challenges

FIGURE 6.2

ALLIED HEALTH PROFESSIONAL COMPETENCY EVALUATION

ANP, APRN, CNS, CCP, FNP, Midwife, NP, NNP, PA, Psychologist (CONT.)

Competency	Required Skill	Met	Not Met	Comment
		Evaluation		
Interpersonal & Communication Skills	Accurately conveys relevant information to patients, families, and colleagues			
	Respects patient confidentiality, privacy, and autonomy			
	Listens effectively			
Professionalism	Is respectful of all members of the healthcare team			
	Demonstrates ethically sound practices			
	Is sensitive to cultural, age, gender, disability issues			
Systems-Based Practice	Understands interaction of their responsibilities with the larger process			
	Is aware of the need for cost-effective care			

The above-stated Allied Health Professional is under my direct supervision. I have completed the above Ongoing Professional Practice Evaluation and indicated the practitioner's overall performance for each of the expectations.

Compliance with expectations was made through retrospective chart review, concurrent chart review, concurrent observation, and/or discussion with other individuals involved in the care of patients.

In addition, I have reviewed the attached privileges and agree that the practitioner continues to be clinically competent to perform the privileges granted.

_____

Sponsoring Physician Name Printed

_____

Signature of Sponsoring Physician

_____

Date

Please return with the Peer Reference Questionnaire

Figure 6.3 depicts specialty-specific competencies for the nurse midwife. Whenever appropriate, specialty-specific indicators should be developed as applicable to the discipline in which the APP practices.

The evaluation process for the APP needs to be outlined in a hospital policy specific to the type of APP. The policy should include the guidelines for both initial and ongoing evaluation, as well as the frequency of the evaluation. It may be important to evaluate APPs more often than physicians, which the medical staff services department will need to determine and include in the policy. The medical staff services department may choose to evaluate the APP more frequently because the APP is not the attending of record and is therefore not routinely showing up in patient records. If an APP is part of the care when there is a negative or questionable outcome, it may not be quickly identified that he or she was involved. Having a policy that requires more routine evaluations may provide the added confirmation that all aspects of the care are given the appropriate focus when needed.

The policy (see Figure 6.4) may also include standard and specialty-specific measures. A policy should allow the medical staff services department to make changes as needed, especially during the initial implementation of the evaluation process and as options for data collection improve or change over time.

Conclusion

APPs and the physicians who work with them are valuable resources in the development of assessment measures and processes. The opportunity for continued improvement and refinement of the process will certainly be possible when multiple resources are considered and included.

Returning to the case study presented at the beginning of the chapter, once the medical staff services department was able to determine the appropriate privileging for APPs and the frequency of ongoing evaluation as well as the evaluation tool, they were able to confidently provide the credentials committee with data supporting the APPs and their clinical activity within the facility. It was also recognized that as their facility advanced in the attribution and capturing of APP data, their processes would continue to improve.

FIGURE 6.3
NURSE MIDWIFE PROCTOR REPORT

Date of this review: _____   Medical record number/patient name: _____

Midwife proctored: _____   Proctor's name: _____

Was this a low-risk delivery? ☐ Yes ☐ No   If no, please explain _____

_____

_____

Evaluate in terms of completeness and accuracy	Acceptable	Marginal (please explain)	Unacceptable (please explain)	N/A
Predelivery work-up				
Sponsoring physician notified and physician's name documented in chart at time of admission	☐	☐	☐	☐
H&Ps are complete, accurate, and on chart	☐	☐	☐	☐
Consent(s) are appropriate and signed	☐	☐	☐	☐
Ancillary services are used appropriately	☐	☐	☐	☐
Progress notes are complete and timely	☐	☐	☐	☐
Comments: _____				
OB management				
Predelivery management	☐	☐	☐	☐
Labor management	☐	☐	☐	☐
Anesthesia management	☐	☐	☐	☐
Newborn management	☐	☐	☐	☐
Postdelivery management	☐	☐	☐	☐
Conduct in labor and delivery room	☐	☐	☐	☐
Comments: _____				
Patient management				
Clinical judgment: Degree to which delivery conforms to acceptable practices	☐	☐	☐	☐

FIGURE 6.3
NURSE MIDWIFE PROCTOR REPORT (CONT.)

Evaluate in terms of completeness and accuracy	Acceptable	Marginal (please explain)	Unacceptable (please explain)	N/A
Technical skill:	❏	❏	❏	❏
Complications (if any) are recognized and managed appropriately	❏	❏	❏	❏
Discharge plans (including patient instructions) are reflected in chart	❏	❏	❏	❏
Appropriate collaboration/consultation with or referral to sponsoring physician/group	❏	❏	❏	❏
Comments: _____				
Overall performance				
Interaction with colleagues, staff, and patient	❏	❏	❏	❏
Overall impression of care provided	❏	❏	❏	❏
Comments: _____				

Is there any aspect of this patient's treatment and follow-up with which you are uneasy or uncomfortable?

❏ No ❏ Yes If yes, please explain: _____

_____

Proctor's signature: _____ Date:_____

Please return to the medical staff office immediately following completion.

Source: Mercy Medical Center, Nampa, ID.

 The Medical Staff's Guide to Overcoming Competence Assessment Challenges

---

FIGURE 6.4

PERFORMANCE FEEDBACK PROCESS FOR APPs
(NURSE PRACTITIONERS AND PHYSICIAN ASSISTANTS)

Purpose/scope: The purpose of this process is to monitor performance/competency of APPs to measure and continually improve performance and provide ongoing assessment in a measurable way. The findings will be reported to the board of directors after the first provisional year and at least every other year thereafter.

Background: Physician assistants (PA) and nurse practitioners (NP) are midlevel practitioners at [X] Medical Center and do not function independently in accordance with the hospital's policy. Physician supervision is outlined in the delegation of services agreement/supervising physician agreement on file in the medical staff office.

Guidelines:

A. Provisional Year

   Performance feedback during the provisional year will occur as follows:

   1) Five cases will be reviewed each quarter and the results reported to the department chair.

   2) The supervising physician and department director(s) will be asked to provide an evaluation quarterly. The department chair will be notified of any adverse findings.

   3) At the end of the provisional year, quarterly reports will be compiled and aggregate information will be reported to the department chair, credentials committee, medical executive committee, and the board of directors.

B. Ongoing Evaluation

   After the provisional year, ongoing evaluation will occur as follows:

   1) Cases are screened for peer review indicators. If a midlevel practitioner was involved in a case that is identified for peer review, the midlevel practitioner will be asked to attend the meeting and participate in the peer review.

   2) If a finding is attributed to the midlevel practitioner, the case will be tracked through the peer review system and reported at the time of reappointment.

   3) At the end of each two-year reappointment period, the supervising physician and department director(s) will be asked to provide an evaluation.

   4) The medical staff office will aggregate the information and report to the department chair who will make a recommendation for reappointment to the credentials committee, medical executive committee, and the board of directors.

FIGURE 6.4

PERFORMANCE FEEDBACK PROCESS FOR APPs
(NURSE PRACTITIONERS AND PHYSICIAN ASSISTANTS) (CONT.)

Measures: Performance evaluation during the provisional year will cover the following dimensions of performance: technical quality, service quality, patient safety, resource utilization, peer and coworker relationships, and citizenship.

The following indicators will be used to measure provider performance against the dimensions of performance. (Indicators in **bold** will be collected by the performance improvement department. Other indicators will be evidenced through an evaluation tool completed by department directors/supervising physician):

A. Technical Quality

   1) **Case volumes by diagnosis/Diagnosis-related group**

   2) **Readmission rates**

   3) **Complication rates**

   4) **Number of cases sent to peer review**

   5) **Mortality rates**

   6) **Number/types of incident reports**

   7) Skills for scope of practice requested/practices within scope

   8) Physician oversight

B. Service Quality

   1) How well providers deliver care to their patients

   2) Use of scripting/participation in other customer service initiatives

   3) Approach/rapport with patients and families

   4) Appropriate communication with the healthcare team

   5) Responding to pages/requests in a timely manner

   6) Timeliness and accuracy of dictation/medical record completion

C. Patient Safety

   1) **Legible, complete, timely, and accurate medical records**

   2) **Use of prohibited abbreviations**

   3) Compliance with universal precautions/hand hygiene

     The Medical Staff's Guide to Overcoming Competence Assessment Challenges

FIGURE 6.4

**PERFORMANCE FEEDBACK PROCESS FOR APPs
(NURSE PRACTITIONERS AND PHYSICIAN ASSISTANTS) (CONT.)**

   D. Resource Utilization

       1) Under-/over-utilization of medications/equipment

       2) Number of denials

       3) Number of avoidable days

   E. Peer and Coworker Relationships

       1) Mutual respect among the heathcare team

       2) Interpersonal relationships/cooperation with other disciplines

       3) Number of complaints

       4) Identifies themselves as PA/NP

       5) Wears a name badge in the facility

   F. Citizenship

       1) Attends meetings when a peer review case is discussed

       2) Maintains patient confidentiality

       3) Supports the mission/vision of the hospital

Source: Mercy Medical Center, Nampa, ID.

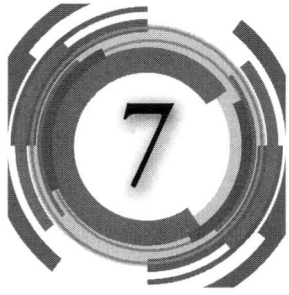

How to Manage the Expanding Role of APPs

Sally Pelletier, CPMSM, CPCS

Dr. Nerv System, a neurosurgeon at Memorial Medical Center, has mentioned in passing to the department chair of surgery that he is training his physician assistant (PA), Ms. Kno Limitations, to do ventriculostomies and to place tong traction and halo fixation devices. Dr. System states that his PA has excellent technique and that Ms. Limitations is permitted this privilege under licensure, which allows the PA to do whatever the physician is privileged to do.

Although the surgery department chair knows that Memorial embraces the benefits that come with the utilization of advanced practice professionals (APP), such as PAs and advanced practice registered nurses (APRN), he questions such a casual mention by Dr. System that this type of training is occuring. He explains to Dr. System that he would like him to put a hold on any further training so that he may investigate whether the hospital has any established protocols to manage this type of training for APPs. He states he will get back to Dr. System within a day or two.

The surgery chair contacts the manager of the medical staff services department. He learns there is no policy regarding physicians training their PAs to do procedures. The chair also asks what the ongoing professional practice evaluation (OPPE) findings had been regarding Ms. Limitations. He learned that although PAs are included in the OPPE process because they are granted clinical privileges, there is little to no performance measurement data on Ms. Limitations or other PAs. However, to their recollection, no issues had been identified related to Ms. Limitations' competence. Review of the PA privilege form reveals that although "assisting at surgery" is certainly included, the procedures referenced by Dr. System are not. Review of the PA state licensure requirements also reveals that PAs are allowed to do whatever the supervising physician delegates as long as the physician is privileged to perform the procedure.

As they continued their discussion, the manager notes that just last week, she had brought to the medicine department chair's attention that PAs were being allowed to do lumbar punctures in the emergency department (ED), even though they did not have that privilege on their current privilege form. Because the medicine chair knew that current competence must be established before granting clinical privileges and that it would be inconsistent to grant a privilege before such competence has been established, she concluded that training PAs to perform lumbar punctures on the job must be okay.

Based on their discussion, the surgery chair and the manager of the medical staff services department realize they needed to further explore how to manage APPs' expanding roles. The manager agreed to bring it to the attention of the credentials committee chair so that the topic could be placed on the agenda.

The topic has come before the credentials committee for consideration. What should the credentials committee do?

Perhaps your organization is struggling with the same issue. Have you ever asked the following questions?

- Do we adequately address our APPs' expanding skills or scopes of practice?

- Are APPs allowed to expand privileges through on-site training?

- Have APPs expanded their scope of privileges without authorization (i.e., "scope creep")?

- What type of education and communication needs to be implemented so that the supervising physicians and the APPs that they supervise are aware of the need to follow a process?

Training Up

APPs (PAs and advanced practice registered nurses [APRN]) who are providing a medical level of care must be privileged through the medical staff process. APRNs are defined by the boards of registered nursing in most states as including the following disciplines:

- Certified nurse midwives (CNM)

- Clinical nurse specialists (CNS)

 The Medical Staff's Guide to Overcoming Competence Assessment Challenges

- Certified registered nurse anesthetists (CRNA)

- Nurse practitioners (NP)

The elements related to the privileging process must be applied regardless of whether the PAs and APRNs are employed by the organization. For example, some NPs may enter the organization via an employment relationship with a physician; others may be employed by the organization. Both groups need to be privileged, the same way that a physician employed or under contract with the hospital must be credentialed and privileged to provide clinical services.

The presence of APPs in hospitals has grown exponentially during the past decade. Collaborating and supervising physicians have realized the value of APPs and often seek to expand the role of APPs. Furthermore, APPs seek to increase their knowledge and skill base and thus their scope of practice. The pending physician shortage provides further incentive for organizations to create mechanisms to expand privileges for APPs. Academic hospitals inherently have a framework in place for on-site education and training. However, in community hospitals that are not teaching institutions, this is not typically the case.

Often, once an organization recognizes that so-called "training up" (physicians training APPs to take on expanded roles) is occurring, the medical staff and administration think of privileging first and foremost. However, privileging is not the first step in this process. The first step in this process must be that the healthcare organization's leadership (governing body, senior administration, and medical staff) determines whether its mission and culture support expansion of privileges for APPs through on-site education and training.

Answers to the following questions will affect this decision:

1. Does the organization's current culture support training up of APPs from both the governing body and medical staff perspectives?

2. Does the hospital's liability carrier allow training up? Is the activity covered by the hospital's policy?

3. If the organization ultimately permits training up, will patient consent be obtained?

Developing a training-up policy

Once the decision is made to offer APPs the opportunity to train up, the organization is now ready to determine the policy and procedures necessary to accomplish this goal. Policy considerations should include the following:

- A purpose statement or objective: The organization must make certain that patient safety and quality are adequately protected by establishing a safe and effective training process to increase the competencies (cognitive and procedural) of each APP who requests additional clinical privileges for which he or she has limited or no training or experience.

- Acknowledgment that APPs who do not meet established eligibility criteria and cannot demonstrate the requisite competence for the requested expansion of privileges may be allowed to train up through privileges granted under the direct supervision of their collaborating or supervising physician or designee. Direct supervision means that the collaborating or supervising physician or designee is acting as a preceptor and is therefore required to be physically present during training and procedures. Precepting is a process through which a practitioner gains experience and/or training on new skills and knowledge. (Note: Proctoring confirms previously acquired competence. Precepting and proctoring are therefore not interchangeable terms.)

- Reference to existing processes for granting clinical privileges: The request for privileges will be considered in accordance with the medical staff bylaws and policies and procedures related to clinical privileging, such as department chair or section chief review and recommendation (if applicable), credentials committee review and recommendation (if applicable), medical executive committee (MEC) review and recommendation, and governing body action.

- Recognition that although the APP may not be able to demonstrate competence for the additional procedures being requested, he or she must meet a certain minimum threshold criteria to even be considered for the train-up privilege. For example, a PA seeking to be trained up in additional procedures for neurosurgery should already meet the following requirements:

  - The governing body's current minimum threshold criteria for education through completion of an Accreditation Review Commission on Education for the Physician Assistant–approved program

  - Current certification by the National Commission on Certification of Physician Assistants

The Medical Staff's Guide to Overcoming Competence Assessment Challenges

- Current licensure to practice as a PA

- Requisite professional liability insurance coverage

- Experience as a first assist in neurosurgery procedures, such as craniotomies and spinal procedures

- For privileges for which there is no established criteria for the APP (e.g., the privilege or procedure was previously only granted to physicians), the governing body must determine whether it will allow APPs to perform the particular privilege or procedure in question. If the answer is no, then no criteria need to be developed. If the answer is yes, then criteria must be developed in accordance with established medical staff policy.

- A procedure for obtaining patient consent for any invasive procedures being performed by an APP under direct supervision or a preceptorship.

This process may seem foreign to some physicians, as it is common for them to continuously train the APP to perform additional procedures and expand the care, treatment, and services that they provide. Therefore, the medical staff must communicate with and educate the supervising physicians and the APPs about the process of training up. The medical staff services department will be a tremendous aid in supporting this process by defining the procedure for the APPs and their collaborating or supervising physician to follow. This procedure should include a written request submitted by the collaborating or supervising physician to train an APP (the physician preceptor[s] must have the privilege[s] being requested by the APP). The request should include:

1. The specific privilege(s) requested

2. The name(s) of preceptor(s)

3. The anticipated length of training

4. Competence measures

5. Patient population (if applicable)

Figure 7.1 is an example of a training-up privilege request form.

FIGURE 7.1

ADVANCED PRACTICE PROFESSIONALS – TRAIN-UP REQUEST FORM

Date of application: _____

Requesting physician: _____

Name of advanced practice professional: _____

Specific privileges being requested under direct supervision: _____
_____

Patient population (if applicable): _____

Name of preceptor(s): _____

Competency measures

_____   _____

_____   _____

_____   _____

_____   _____

Anticipated length of training: _____

Other comments:

_____
_____
_____

_____   _____
Signature – Requesting physician   Date

_____   _____
Signature – Requesting APP   Date

The Medical Staff's Guide to Overcoming Competence Assessment Challenges

It is also important to note that these train-up privileges (under a preceptor) are not time limited, meaning that once the training is completed and the APP wishes to request independent practice privileges, and the collaborating or supervising physician confirms that the APP is competent to perform the privileges independently, then the medical staff policy for modification of clinical privileges should be followed. (Independent practice in this case references that the period of precepting is completed. The APP is still supervised in accordance with organizational policy and state law.)

Once the initial privileging process is complete for the independent practice of the procedure, the privileged APP follows the same path as a privileged physician. The same expectations regarding competence assessment or periodic appraisal apply to the privileged APP (e.g., focused professional practice evaluation [FPPE] and OPPE for Joint Commission–accredited facilities). These expectations are a frequent obstacle for medical staffs and hospitals. Over the past few years, medical staffs have dedicated significant effort to designing and implementing ongoing performance monitoring for physicians. However, less attention has been paid to evaluating the competence of privileged APPs. Nevertheless, the same standards do apply to the privileged APP. Involving these practitioners in the development of measurement standards is the key to moving forward quickly and effectively. See Chapter 6 for tips on assessing APP competence.

TRAINING UP IS AN OPTION FOR SOME PHYSICIANS

Whenever a practitioner who is currently privileged at an organization wishes to increase his or her knowledge and skill base and thus broaden his or her scope of practice, the organization can assist the practitioner by providing the necessary training via a preceptorship program. With physician shortages affecting many healthcare organizations, developing a preceptor policy and process to "train up" current practitioners, such as APPs and physicians, can help meet increasing patient care demands.

The first step is for the organization's applicable leadership (e.g., nursing leaders, the MEC, and board) to determine whether they support the request to implement an on-site education and training process or program. One aspect to consider in a nonacademic medical center is to confirm that the organization's professional liability carrier includes this activity.

Second, once the decision is made to support an education initiative, the organization should develop a clear policy and procedure to ensure that an effective training process is implemented. The training should provide the necessary hands-on education and experience while making certain that patient safety and quality patient care are preserved.

Third, the organization needs to create a policy to support and guide the process. The policy should include, but not be limited to, the following:

TRAINING UP IS AN OPTION FOR SOME PHYSICIANS (CONT.)

- The specific level of supervision required for a preceptor program. The medical staff reviews and grants privileges related to the preceptor program as appropriate.

- The level of supervision that must be provided by a preceptor prior to the clinical privileges being granted.

- An outline of the minimum threshold criteria for allowing preceptorship. If criteria for a preceptorship program have not been established, the medical staff indicates what the process is to evaluate a request. Criteria for privileges, including privileges that require supervision via a preceptor, should be developed as outlined in the medical staff policies.

- Definitions of the different levels of supervision allowed by your organization (i.e., direct, immediately available, indirect, etc.).

- A requirement that the supervising preceptor must currently hold the clinical privileges that the physician requesting a preceptorship wishes to earn.

- A requirement that all requests outline anticipated length of training and competence measures.

Once a practitioner has completed the preceptor process and has met all required competence measures, the practitioner should then submit a request for additional privileges, which must be granted separately before he or she can independently perform those privileges.

Revisiting Memorial Medical Center

Let's revisit our question from the beginning of this chapter.

What should the credentials committee do?

1. The first step is to put a moratorium on the request to determine the hospital's (i.e., governing body's) position on the training up of APPs.

2. Second, the credentials committee should communicate with Dr. System (and others, such as the medicine chair) that the organization needs to determine the proper steps to follow as outlined in this chapter. If the governing body decides to allow APPs to expand privileges through on-site

training, and the professional liability carrier is in agreement, then the credentials committee can develop a policy to adequately address the expanding skills or scope of practice of APPs. The policy will then be communicated via established medical staff channels so that the supervising physicians and the APPs that they supervise are aware of the need to follow a process.

3. Third, Dr. System should then request in writing to the medical staff services department that Ms. Kno Limitations be able to train up to perform ventriculostomies and to place tong traction and halo fixation devices while he serves as the preceptor. He should also provide the anticipated length of training, appropriate competence measures, and the patient population (if applicable).

4. The request for privileges under direct supervision will be considered in accordance with the medical staff bylaws and policies and procedures related to clinical privileging, e.g., department chair review and recommendation (if applicable), credentials committee review and recommendation (if applicable), MEC review and recommendation, and governing body action.

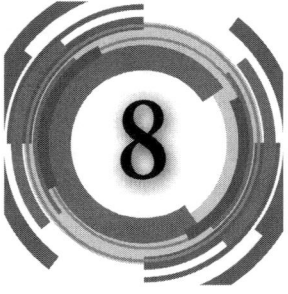

8 Assessing the Competence of Telemedicine Practitioners

Carol S. Cairns, CPMSM, CPCS

CASE STUDY

Saint Elsewhere is about to sign a five-year contract with Teleradiology of America (TRA). TRA is a large, international company serving hundreds of hospitals with a cadre of several hundred radiologists. According to the contract, TRA will begin interpreting radiology exams from 10:00 p.m. to 6:00 a.m. seven days per week, 30 days after signing the contract.

As an afterthought, the CEO of Saint Elsewhere has come to Sally Problem-Solver, director of the medical staff services department, to notify her of the pending contract and to ask whether there were any issues that needed to be identified and resolved. The CEO stated that the contract radiologists were fully supportive of this concept and, in fact, had suggested it. The CEO stated he had also spoken to the chief of staff and had gained her support as well.

What should Sally Problem-Solver do? What aspects of the new contract need to be evaluated? Who else needs to be involved in the discussions?

Sally should start by asking for a week to evaluate the contract, assess the credentialing and privileging requirements as related to the provision of teleradiology services, talk to the medical staff leaders, and then respond to the CEO.

Sally points out to the CEO that there may be significant medical, legal, and compliance issues to be evaluated. Therefore, to protect patients and the hospital, further review of the contract and new service should be done prior to TRA providing services. Some immediate areas of concern include the following:

- How many of the hundreds of radiologists will need to be credentialed and privileged for the service to be provided? (Currently, the medical staff services department is understaffed by one full-time equivalent due to a hiring freeze.)

- Do the credentialing/privileging criteria of the teleradiology service match the criteria in the medical staff bylaws?

- Are the credentialing verification processes of the teleradiology service equivalent to those of St. Elsewhere?

- How will the focused professional practice evaluation (FPPE) and ongoing professional practice evaluation (OPPE) be conducted?

- Are revisions necessary to the current radiology privilege form to accommodate the exercise of radiology privileges through a telemedicine mechanism?

Lastly, Sally informs the CEO that under current bylaws and accreditation requirements, these radiologists would not qualify for temporary privileges for patient care need. The current radiology group was providing sufficient coverage, and thus the definition of patient care need would not be met.

Although a bit frustrated, the CEO acknowledges that these are important issues he had not sufficiently considered. He agrees to a one-week delay in the process and schedules a meeting with Sally to follow up.

Introducing a Telemedicine Service at Your Facility

Healthcare has seen an explosion in technology over the past two decades, making possible diagnostic and therapeutic approaches to clinical care previously only seen in science fiction movies. These advances bring new challenges to overcome, questions to answer, solutions to craft, processes to establish, and policies to develop. Chapter 10 outlines the issues related to introducing new technology into an organization.

The clear answer to the case study given above is to have an organizational policy that addresses the introduction of new technology, services, and/or procedures and then follow that policy, as applicable, to the introduction of teleradiology services.

Because St. Elsewhere lacks such a policy, the organization needs to step back, develop a policy, and apply the policy as the facility considers the introduction of teleradiology services to support patient care.

This case study outlines the concept of a significant change in care delivery. Because several hundred radiologists work for TRA, St. Elsewhere may need to privilege a significant number of off-site radiologists to provide teleradiology services. Despite the complexity of this task, requests for privileges to deliver patient care through telemedicine may be less complex than contemplating a significant change in clinical services.

For example, a consulting psychiatrist may be privileged to provide care within an organization and wants permission to provide assessment and counseling services through a telemedicine link. In this case, the medical staff and board may determine that the telemedicine link is just a different way to provide the same service that the psychiatrist provides on-site. There is no need to apply the steps related to new technology or new services. This example, then, begs the question, "What is telemedicine?"

Defining Telemedicine

According to the American Telemedicine Association, telemedicine is defined as the use of medical information exchanged from one site to another via electronic communications to improve patients' health status. Telemedicine is a subcategory of telehealth.

> To differentiate the site of the practitioner from the location of service to the patient, regulators and accreditors have coined the following terms:
>
> - "Distant site" describes the location of the practitioner
>
> - "Originating site" describes the location of the patient and facility receiving the service

Telemedicine takes many forms and has many clinical applications. In some applications of telemedicine, the clinical effect is immediate, particularly in therapeutic modalities; in some other applications of telemedicine, the clinical effect is delayed, particularly in diagnostic modalities, such as teleradiology.

Examples of telemedicine, clinical uses, and its effect on the patient include the following:

Teleradiology

Teleradiology is currently the most common form of telemedicine. Radiological images are transmitted to a radiologist at a "distant site" and interpreted quickly, with resultant opinions available for patient diagnosis and treatment. Generally, teleradiology services supplement the on-site radiologists by providing interpretations during evening hours and weekends. Thereafter, the on-site radiologist commonly overreads the images and renders a final interpretation.

In some healthcare facilities, the teleradiologists' interpretations are rendered from the distant site 24 hours per day, seven days per week, and are considered the final read.

Some organizations seek teleradiology consultations in areas of specific expertise, such as neurologic radiology or pediatric radiology.

Telepsychiatry, telepsychology, and telecounseling

Telepsychiatry, telepsychology, and telecounseling are further examples of common forms of telemendicine. The combination of current technology and this specific clinical specialty make delivery of these clinical services quite easy. Telemedicine allows easy access to these clinical services by patients who may otherwise need to travel significant distances for those services or whose medical condition makes on-site access much more problematic. An additional benefit is that delivery of mental health services via telemedicine also increases patient privacy in this sensitive field. Patients are able to access mental health services in the privacy of their homes (or other confidential environment) and thus avoid "being seen" in the office of a psychiatrist, psychologist, or counselor.

According to the Veterans Administration, there is a remarkable increase in the need for mental health services for returning armed services veterans who have a variety of mental health needs. Soldiers are returning with posttraumatic brain injuries, posttraumatic stress disorders, and other complications. One solution to meeting the demand is telehealth.

Another common example of delivery of mental health services via telemedicine is within the prison system, where there is a significant clinical need for behavioral health services. However, the prison setting poses challenges to practitioner safety and requires additional time and resources to deliver the needed therapy. Therefore, prisons have utilized telemedicine to increase access to these services.

Electronic intensive care services (E-ICU)

E-ICU is another application of telemedicine. The delivery of this service is generally characterized by a contractual arrangement between the hospital and/or system with a group of physicians specializing in providing care to intensive care patients. The service is provided from one (or more) remote sites. Each remote site mirrors the ICU patient monitoring system in each contracted hospital ICU along with visual and auditory contact with individual patients. The E-ICU physician remotely manages the patient according to the terms of the contract.

Cardiology and neurology

Cardiology or neurology tracings may be interpreted through use of telemetry. Some organizations have contracted for remote readings of electrocardiograms and/or electroencephalograms. Some are for all readings, some are for focused specialty areas (e.g., pediatric), and some may be needed only for times of coverage for an absent practitioner(s).

Specialty/subspecialty consultation

Specialty and subspecialty consultation may be provided by telemedicine. Healthcare organizations that have limited availability or access to consultative services can utilize a camera, nurse, and an examination room to provide expanded services on a practitioner's order.

Intraoperative neurodiagnostic services

Intraoperative neurodiagnostic services are now expanding with the capabilities of telemonitoring. Services are provided off-site by neurologists, nurse practitioners, and neurodiagnostic technicians.

As technology continues to advance, physician shortages increase, and cost containment efforts intensify, there will be an ever-expanding opportunity to provide broader and more comprehensive services through the use of telemedicine technology.

Who Provides Telemedicine Services?

Telemedicine services are provided in a number of ways. For example, teleradiology is provided by large and small physician-owned groups. Some of these groups provide care on a local, regional, or national basis. Services are even provided from international locations to take advantage of time zone differences.

Another supplier is an individual hospital that provides teleradiology services to other hospitals. For example, the largest hospital within a system might provide teleradiology services to one or more smaller hospitals within that same system.

Another supplier might be the individual practitioner(s) who agrees to provide electrocardiogram or electroencephalogram interpretations or specialty consultations to the hospital.

Requirements of Regulators and Accreditation Agencies

The affect of telemedicine on healthcare delivery is demonstrated by the current Centers for Medicare & Medicaid Services (CMS) *Conditions of Participation* (*CoP*). In July 2011, CMS published new credentialing standards that focused on the clinical delivery of care utilizing telemedicine. Prior to that date, the only mention in the standards regarding telemedicine practitioners related to licensure requirements. (The telemedicine practitioner must have a valid license in the state where the hospital is and patients are receiving care.)

In the July 2011 revision, CMS placed great emphasis on telemedicine by adding ten-plus pages to the *CoP* in three areas of the medical staff standards (CMS *CoP* standards §482.12[a][8] Standard: Medical Staff, §482.22[a][3-4] Standard: Composition of the Medical Staff, and §482.22[c][6] Standard: Medical Staff Bylaws). Essentially, all of the new standards are related to the credentialing and privileging of telemedicine practitioners. The additions to the *CoP* include new standards, interpretive guidelines, and survey procedures outlining expectations and processes specific to telemedicine.

Once again, it is important to note that these telemedicine standards apply not only to physicians and dentists but also to advanced practice professionals (APP) as well.

Following publication of these new standards, each accrediting agency also made modifications to their respective standards. It is important for each healthcare facility to be cognizant of the requirements of all applicable regulators and/or accreditors for their specific organization.

Effect of Telemedicine Regulations

The telemedicine standards are quite complex and must be clearly understood by the organization's governing body, senior management, and medical staff leaders.

In summary, some of the more important aspects of the CMS telemedicine standards include the following:

- If the telemedicine services are provided by a distant-site hospital or telemedicine entity, there is a written agreement between the distant site and the healthcare organization that is receiving the telemedicine services that outlines all required aspects of the telemedicine service. This agreement specifies the obligation of the distant site to ensure that practitioners are credentialed and privileged in compliance with CMS regulations for telemedicine practitioners.

- Each telemedicine practitioner must be granted site-specific privileges by the healthcare facility that is receiving telemedicine services. In accordance with CMS regulations, there are essentially three options to grant privileges to telemedicine practitioners, highlighted below.

Apply existing credentialing and privileging processes

The governing body may elect to apply existing credentialing and privileging processes to the telemedicine practitioner. Thus, the current medical staff processes prevail as outlined in the medical staff governance documents and apply to telemedicine practitioners. In this instance, the medical staff should evaluate whether all verification processes are applicable and necessary for the telemedicine practitioner. For example, if an organization routinely confirms all previous affiliations and requires a competence assessment from each facility for every applicant, this may be a very onerous standard for telemedicine practitioners, as well as the medical staff services department.

An appropriate alternative might be to create a policy that shares responsibility and accountability with the contracting telemedicine entity to verify the telemedicine practitioners' work history. For example, if a tele-radiologist provides interpretation to 30 healthcare facilities, the hospital may ask the practitioner to identify five facilities where he or she does the majority of his or her work. This information could be then verified by the medical staff services department using the usual documents and processes. The medical staff services department could then request that the telemedicine entity verifies the remaining information through a single letter globally addressing the practitioner's performance in all practice locations.

An excellent practice is for the hospital to require that the agreement with the telemedicine entity specify that the hospital will be provided all information regarding the practitioner—including negative information and complaints. By specifying this expectation, the hospital notifies the entity that it wants to review all information known to the telemedicine entity. Further, the hospital wishes to retain the responsibility of evaluating the information received and not delegate that obligation to the telemedicine entity.

Utilize existing credentials verification process or data collected by the telemedicine agency, or both

The governing body may elect to utilize existing credentials verification processes, credentials verification data collected by the telemedicine agency, or a combination of both. The medical staff bases its privileging recommendation to the governing body on the collected information.

Caution: If a hospital chooses to delegate the credentialing verification process to the telemedicine entity, the medical staff must evaluate whether the telemedicine entity uses a process equivalent to that of the medical staff services department. In other words, the information requested and received from the telemedicine entity should be comparable to that requested/received by the hospital for other applicants.

Act on medical staff recommendations that rely on credentialing and privileging decisions from the distant site

The governing body may elect to consider hospital medical staff recommendations that rely on the credentialing and privileging decisions pertaining to practitioners utilized by the distant-site hospital or telemedicine entity. (The practitioner must be employed by or utilized by the distant-site hospital or entity.)

The distant site must provide a current listing of all practitioners covered by the agreement, including privileges, at the distant site. The hospital has evidence of internal review of the services rendered and provides feedback to the distant site. The distant site includes that feedback in the periodic evaluation of the practitioner. At minimum, the hospital must review and report all adverse events and complaints.

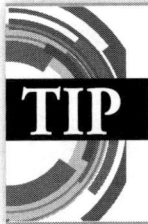

> **TIP**
>
> As organizations evaluate the three options mentioned, every effort should be made to utilize appropriate credentialing verification documents from the telemedicine hospital or entity. This decision should be outlined in the contractual agreement, reduce duplicative efforts, costs, turnaround time, and resource consumption.

If an organization chooses the second or third option, documentation for each applicant should reflect whether the medical staff conducted its own review or relied on the decisions of the distant site hospital or telemedicine entity.

Privileging Telemedicine Practitioners

Organizations should not make the task of creating specialty-specific telemedicine privileges difficult. The process should begin with reviewing the existing privilege form for the specialty. The form should be modified to include a section for telemedicine privileges that would reflect only those privileges that apply to utilizing telemedicine technology.

Figure 8.1 is an excerpt of an example of how a site-specific, criterion-based, core privileging form for radiology has been quickly and simply modified to include a core privilege for telemedicine physicians. (Please note that the entire radiology core privileging form can be found in *Core Privileges for Physicians, Fifth Edition*, published by HCPro and available at *www.hcmarketplace.com*.)

FIGURE 8.1

CORE TELERADIOLOGY PRIVILEGES

❏ **Requested:** Perform general diagnostic radiology (x-ray, radionuclides, ultrasound, and electromagnetic radiation) to diagnose diseases of patients of all ages via a teleradiography link. Responsible for communicating critical values and critical findings consistent with medical staff policy. The core privileges in this specialty include the interpretations on the attached list and such other interpretations that are extensions of the same techniques and skills.

Criteria: The same as for the diagnostic radiology core.

Teleradiology

To the applicant: If you wish to exclude any interpretations, please strike through the interpretations that you do not wish to request, and then initial and date.

- Computed tomography (CT) of the head, neck, spine, body, chest ([including/excluding] cardiac), abdomen, pelvis, and extremities and their associated vasculatures

- Diagnostic nuclear radiology of the head, neck, spine, body, chest (including the heart), abdomen, pelvis, and extremities and their associated vasculatures

- Magnetic resonance imaging (MRI) of the head, neck, spine, body, chest ([including/excluding] cardiac), abdomen, pelvis, extremities and their associated vasculatures, and muscular skeletal structures, etc.

- Positron emission tomography (PET)

- Mammography (in accordance with Mammography Quality System Regulation [MQSR] required qualifications)

- Routine imaging (e.g., interpretation of plain films)

Competence Assessment Unique to Telemedicine

Essentially, assessing competence for telemedicine practitioners does not differ from the processes utilized in the acute care setting. The same requirements and expectations outlined throughout this book are applied to the delivery of care through telemedicine. It does not matter what terms are used by the medical staff and the organization to describe the competence assessment function, such as performance monitoring, performance improvement, quality assessment, quality improvement, OPPE, FPPE, peer review, etc.

Most measurement indicators and benchmark rates apply to telemedicine practitioners. The process of evaluating care should essentially mirror the medical staff process as outlined within the medical staff bylaws, policies and procedures, and the performance improvement plan. The only addition would be to determine whether the outcome will also be reported to the telemedicine entity, depending on which approval process is selected. (See "Effect of Telemedicine Requirements" earlier in this chapter.)

Once again, it is important to use processes that are already in place and keep things as simple as possible. For example, in many organizations, the teleradiology interpretation is considered a preliminary read. The following morning, the on-site radiologist overreads all films/images. If this is the routine, this effort reflects peer review of 100% of the teleradiologists' work. Thus all that is needed is a mechanism to capture the outcome and report to appropriate parties.

Sample indicators for review of performance of a radiologist are included in Figure 8.2.

FIGURE 8.2
SAMPLE INDICATORS FOR RADIOLOGIST PERFORMANCE REVIEW

Medical Staff Department	Indicator	Type Rate Review Rule	Excellent Target	Acceptable Target
Radiology	Average report turnaround time for radiology services subcategorized by routine and complex cases and service type	Rate	95% <6 hrs Inp <12 hrs OP	85% <12 hrs Inp <24 hrs OP
Radiology	CT stroke turnaround time frame - CT order → Dictated within 45 minutes	Rate	95%	85%
Radiology	Random case radiology interpretation correlation category 3 or 4	Rate	2%	5%
Radiology	Suspicious mammography findings confirmed by breast biopsy	Rate	NA	25-40%

Privileged and Confidential under the Illinois Medical Study Act
NA-Not Applicable

 The Medical Staff's Guide to Overcoming Competence Assessment Challenges

These indicators are no different for the teleradiologist. Outcome measures are compared with those of the other practitioners within the radiology service (regardless of whether they are on-site or off-site).

Evaluation parameters of the consulting psychiatrist (per the example earlier in this chapter) would be the same for services rendered via telemetry. If the psychiatrist is providing services only via telemetry and there are no other psychiatrists available to evaluate the care he or she provides, then it is the responsibility of the medical staff to establish a mechanism to evaluate the care. Chapter 9 provides solutions to this issue.

If the clinical services are provided by a defined external entity as opposed to a single individual (e.g., group of radiologists, contracted E-ICU physicians, multispecialty group, etc.), the hospital and its medical staff could require as part of the contract that peer review be done in accordance with the requirements of the organization's regulator or accreditor as appropriate. Further, the hospital could require that all results of all telemedicine practitioners with privileges be shared with the hospital and interpreted by the medical staff.

> **Note:** The external telemedicine entity must share performance monitoring/improvement activities with the contracting hospital if the organization's governing body chooses the option to consider hospital medical staff recommendations that rely on the credentialing and privileging decisions pertaining to practitioners utilized by of the distant-site hospital or telemedicine entity. (The practitioner must be employed by or utilized by the distant-site hospital or entity.)

Some telehealth practitioners may provide services infrequently at the originating facility. Chapter 11 provides helpful options for evaluating competence.

Evaluation of Telemedicine by Specialty

As noted in the beginning of this chapter, there are many ways that telemedicine may enable the delivery of medical care. One can only imagine what the future will bring in this regard. It is important that organizations establish a routine process to evaluate changes in healthcare and routinely follow the established process. The case study at the beginning of this chapter highlighted what can happen when an organization does not have such a process in place.

Due to the complexity and various options allowed regarding credentialing and privileging telemedicine services, it is important for organizations to create policies/procedures applicable to each specialty. For example, in the case study, St. Elsewhere may choose the second option to credential and privilege all teleradiologists.

The governing body may elect to utilize existing credentialing verification processes, credentialing verification data collected by the telemedicine agency, or a combination of both. The medical staff bases its recommendation to the governing body regarding granting of privileges on the collected information.

However, if the organization chooses to deliver a new E-ICU or telepsychiatry service, the organization may choose the first option of completing all credentialing and privileging processes on-site and utilizing existing policies. Organizations should refrain from approaching the delivery of care in the same way for every specialty.

Revisiting St. Elsewhere

As we return to St. Elsewhere, we find that the CEO (wisely!) agreed with the request of Sally Problem-Solver, director of the medical staff services department, to further evaluate the proposed teleradiology contract. Sally had agreed to evaluate the proposed teleradiology contract in relation to credentialing, privileging, and competence assessment, which included review of the regulatory and accreditation requirements. The CEO and Sally had subsequently agreed to meet the following week and invite Dr. Roentgen, the physician director of radiology, and Dr. Barr, the credentials committee chair.

At the follow-up meeting, Sally reported her concerns regarding the immediate signing of the contract. She suggested a short moratorium to evaluate the credentialing, privileging, and competence assessment options as well as those processes utilized by TRA. Sally suggested that St. Elsewhere obtain information from TRA on the following questions:

- Is TRA accredited by The Joint Commission (St. Elsewhere's accrediting agency) under the ambulatory standards?

- What elements and methods of credentials verification does TRA employ?

- What is the general scope of practice for the teleradiologists? How does this compare to the services at St. Elsewhere?

- What assessment measures does TRA use to ensure practitioners are competent?

- What would be the minimum number of teleradiologists assigned to St. Elsewhere? (TRA's literature identified resources of 300-plus radiologists.)

Sally educated Dr. Barr regarding the CMS and Joint Commission requirements for telemedicine practitioners and the effect on the current credentialing, privileging, and competence assessment processes at St. Elsewhere. The credentials chair and Sally then proposed the following process be followed prior to signing a contract with the telemedicine entity.

First, St. Elsewhere would evaluate the efficacy of radiology interpretations via a telemedicine link. This evaluation would include:

- Review of needed equipment and/or staff proficiencies

- Evaluation of medical staff support for this service

- Survey of the experiences of other hospitals utilizing this modality, including some clients of TRA

- Evaluation of the financial effect on the current or future hospital resources

Second, if the evaluation processes described above revealed a green light to move forward, the next steps would be:

- Identify the various credentialing, privileging, and competence assessment options and determine the best option for St. Elsewhere. The resulting recommendation(s) would be forwarded to the governing body.

- Revise the radiology privilege form to include a telemedicine privilege.

- Establish performance measurement standards for teleradiology (e.g., turnaround time, availability for phone consultation regarding interpretations, errors in interpretation adjusted by severity, etc.), as well as designation of responsible parties.

- Identify roots of performance issues and effective ways to manage them.

- Limit the number of privileged teleradiologists to 15 to 20.

- Include pertinent expectations in the written agreement.

Third, the medical staff provides input into the appropriateness of TRA as the teleradiology vendor while the hospital selects TRA or another vendor, revises the contract as appropriate and necessary, and establishes a realistic effective start date.

The CEO and Dr. Roentgen admitted they had been caught off guard by the extent of the issues brought forward. After discussion, they agreed that signing the contract with TRA was premature at this time. The plan outlined by the credentials chair and Sally was approved and responsibilities were assigned.

The CEO and credentials committee chair asked Sally to draft a policy to introduce new technology, services, or procedures for medical staff leaders, senior administration, and the governing body to consider. Next, the CEO asked Sally to be part of future considerations regarding expansion of patient care services at St. Elsewhere. Lastly, the CEO voiced his support to fill the vacant position in the medical staff services department.

9

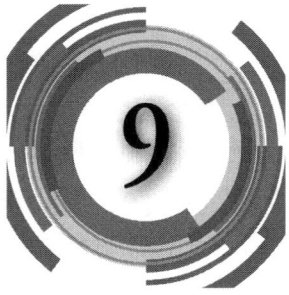

Assessing a Single Practitioner in a Specialty Area

Frances M. Ponsioen, CPMSM, CPCS

CASE STUDY

The credentials committee at Middle of Nowhere Hospital has received an application for a much-needed neurologist. The application includes glowing references and evidence of education and training in some of the best institutions in the country. The administration is shocked but very pleased that they have been able to recruit this neurologist to the area, which has been underserved for quite some time in the area of neurology.

The physician, young, well trained, and experienced, made the decision to relocate to this isolated hospital because he wanted to be closer to his parents and extended aging family. His life decision, while difficult, has benefited the community of Middle of Nowhere Hospital.

The medical staff services department is not quite sure how to handle this application, because (a) it does not have a neurology privilege form, and (b) it is unsure how and by whom this physician will be assessed when there is no other neurologist on staff. The medical services professional (MSP), understanding the need for this physician within the community, accepts the application from the physician and begins the verification process. While processing the application, she works with the credentials committee chair and the department of medicine chair to develop the appropriate neurology privilege form that is setting-specific and contains services and procedures that the hospital can support. She also solicits the applicant's help in developing the form, understanding that he is instrumental in establishing what a qualified neurologist needs to do within a hospital setting.

Hospitals across the country vary widely in how they meet regulatory requirements (e.g., The Joint Commission's focused professional practice evaluation [FPPE] and ongoing professional practice evaluation [OPPE]), making developing a competency assessment process difficult.

The majority of the medical staff members in this small community hospital are family medicine practitioners; the rest are surgeons and subspecialty practitioners. The few specialists on staff are easily assessed by their peers through their current ongoing evaluation process. However, a single practitioner in the specialty of neurology is not typical for this medical staff. How will it assess the physician initially and on an ongoing basis?

The medical staff director and credentials committee chair agreed that through their privileging process, they would be able to assess the initial qualifications of the new physician based on his qualifications to meet predefined eligibility criteria. Primary source verification is standard for all new applicants and includes a thorough investigation of the practitioner's education and training, claims history, previous clinical experience related to the privileges requested, as well as the gathering of recent peer references to provide evidence of current clinical competence. However, they wanted to make sure that they take any additional steps to ensure that the applicant is qualified for the requested privileges, as well as confirm his overall experience and knowledge in neurology.

Determining Competence With No Reference Point

The process for assessing a single practitioner in a specialty should already be in place through established policy and the general data collection already being done on all practitioners regardless of specialty. Using data that are already being collected for the members of the medical staff will be helpful while the medical staff determines indicators for the specific specialty in question. General data elements that assist in a competence assessment include:

- Mortality rates

- Complication rates

- Average length of stay

- Adverse events

- Return to surgery

- Any compliance issues with other metrics that are being measured

     The Medical Staff's Guide to Overcoming Competence Assessment Challenges

Reviewing what is already being collected and then determining what elements pertain to this single specialty will provide a starting point on how to assess the practitioner. In addition to data elements, a retrospective review of patient records will allow the reviewing physician and/or committee to determine whether the practitioner is adhering to hospital policy as it pertains to medical record completion, referrals, and other documentation requirements that all members of the staff are expected to comply with.

In addition to retrospective review, an initial focused assessment or an ongoing assessment may include documented conversations with peers who have worked with the practitioner or observed the practitioner during the assessment period. Initial focused assessments should be timely and over a condensed period of time as pertinent to the particular specialty. Following the initial assessment period, the practitioner moves into an ongoing or "routine" assessment period as established by the organization. Many hospitals find that three eight-month assessment periods work well within a 24-month reappointment cycle. Certain clinical decisions and/or practices will be difficult for other practitioners to assess if they are not in the same specialty, but they should be able to assess at least some clinical decisions (e.g., a general surgeon should be able to assess the basic surgical skills of a plastic or vascular surgeon), as well as interpersonal communication skills and professionalism, which are also important. The suggested methods for assessment can be used during the initial application period as well as on-going assessment and/or evaluation.

In the case of the new neurologist at Middle of Nowhere Hospital, the credentials committee may also request that the practitioner provide additional documentation supporting his or her experience within his or her specialty. Documentation may include a case log, evidence of current activity specific to the privileges being requested, ongoing performance results, and the number of recent procedural cases performed. The activity log or case log should include a supporting letter from the primary facility if the applicant has been out of training for more than one year. The letter and questionnaire form should include the following:

- Questions referencing the six core competencies developed by the American Board of Medical Specialties and the Accreditation Council for Graduate Medical Education and adopted by The Joint Commission

- Attestation to the practitioner's standing and activity within his or her previous institution

- Past or current quality and/or peer review concerns from the previous institution

- A professional reference from the residency program director of the institution where the specialist trained if the practitioner has just recently completed his or her training program in the last five years

As with the new neurologist at Middle of Nowhere Hospital, the medical staff services department should reach out to the practitioner's residency program director to complete a questionnaire referencing the six core competencies. Such a questionnaire will ensure that the key elements required by the credentials committee are addressed, allowing the committee to make a fair assessment of the practitioner. For added confirmation of clinical competence, the medical staff should provide the residency program director with a copy of the privilege form and ask the program director to confirm that the applicant has been appropriately trained for the privileges he or she has requested.

The credentials committee should also elect to contact references and/or the residency program director at the facility where the specialist most recently worked or trained. A phone call will provide not only an opportunity to gather more information but also a more personal assessment that can be reported back to the committee and included in the overall assessment. A personal phone interview with a peer reference will carry a higher weight than the completion of a form letter or questionnaire. A conversation between physician leaders on behalf of the credentialing and privileging process should provide additional insight into the character and behavior of the applicant, which will be helpful to a committee that does not have the specialty in question represented in its membership.

Conducting Ongoing Evaluation of the Specialist

Ongoing review of a single practitioner in a specialty is typically more problematic and should include all suggested methods for initially determining competence, as well as specific data indicators collected through hospital activity. The specialty-specific indicators may be added after the practitioner has completed an initial evaluation period (FPPE) and activity levels have been determined by the credentials committee.

Involving the physician in the development of specialty-specific indicators will be helpful when combined with the organization's own research through specialty societies, associations, and boards. Resources specific to neurology (as in the example at the beginning of this chapter) may include the American Academy of Neurology, American Society of Neuroimaging, and the Society of Vascular and Interventional Neurology.

The credentials committee should also consider alternatives to specialty-specific indicators as a form of assessment. Similar to what was done during the initial assessment period, interviewing other physicians and/or facility staff members who have had an opportunity to work with the specialist will provide valuable insight into the specialist's interpersonal and communication skills and professionalism. By addressing these two core competencies in addition to the limited data and/or specialty indicators, the committee will be in a better position to summarize the assessment and make the appropriate recommendations.

External Reviews

External reviewers should be considered when there is a lack of internal experts and/or resources. The lack of an internal reviewer is not uncommon in a small community hospital, especially when there is only one specialist in a given specialty. An external review, either through a contracted service or a reciprocal agreement with another hospital, may be necessary when specific cases need to be reviewed to determine the ongoing clinical competence of the specialist. External reviews can be done by an agency or a physician within the same specialty who is not a member of the medical staff (and may not even be within the same city or state). A facility may reach out to another organization that can provide the review with the help of a physician within the same specialty.

The completed review report should be handled confidentially and as a protected peer review document in the same manner as all other reviews, which is to say that they are reviewed by the quality and/or credentials committee as part of its ongoing review of all physicians. In this case, the review is being done as part of a routine assessment; the committee or physician reviewing the report may never need to question the findings provided and simply include the results with the overall assessment.

The organization should consider external reviews for benchmarking purposes, especially when there is no internal data available for comparison. Benchmarking data through an external data source will provide the organization and the practitioner with best practices in the specialty area. The physician and organization will be able to use the external review as a baseline for future improvements in quality data as it relates to the specialty.

Providing the physician with the outcome of the external review will not only provide a baseline for future quality improvements, but will also give the physician some assurance that he or she is being assessed by a peer within his or her specialty. If any comments and/or recommendations are made as a result of the review, the practitioner will know that they are being made by a peer with the same level of training and experience. It's important to remember that the external review is typically needed only when there is a need for an evaluation of technical competence. In most cases, any physician serving on a quality or credentials committee will be able to easily evaluate a physician in areas of communication, interpersonal skills, or recordkeeping.

As mentioned earlier in this chapter, the softer skills (e.g., interpersonal skills, record keeping, professionalism, communication) may be assessed by other practitioners or even other non-physician members of the healthcare team. It is only when a matter of technical skill or clinical knowledge arises that an external peer within the same discipline can prove invaluable.

Good collaboration with internal and external sources has provided the medical staff services department and physician leadership at Middle of Nowhere Hospital with options for a successful assessment process. Determining what works best for the organization and the practitioner will be their final step. However, it is certainly expected that as each assessment period is completed, changes and/or improvements should be considered. As the physician becomes more active within the facility, the assessment process will potentially change. Middle of Nowhere Hospital can now provide neurology services to the community. The work that has been done to develop an appropriate assessment process has better prepared them for any other specialists relocating to their facility.

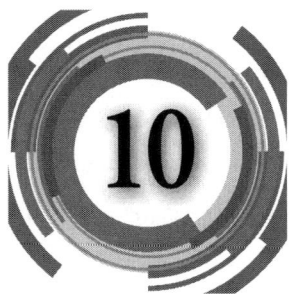

New Technology, Services, and Procedures

Anne Roberts, CPCS, CPMSM

A large medical center has opened a second hospital. Dr. Patella, an orthopedic surgeon, has submitted a request to perform spine surgery at the new facility. He currently holds privileges to perform spine surgery at the main campus. He has requested to start scheduling patients immediately at the new location, and administration is excited to begin offering expanded services in the new market. The medical staff services department has received the request from Dr. Patella for additional privileges.

The medical staff services department needs to determine whether the medical staff and the governing body are prepared to offer spine services at the new facility. When reviewing the privilege delineations for the new site, that particular group of privileges was not included in the initial list. The medical services professional (MSP) contacts the orthopedic surgery division chief and the chief of surgery to discuss the request and discovers that they do not feel that the new facility is prepared to offer spine procedures.

The division chief has indicated that he will be denying the request for additional privileges; however, the MSP advises that because the privileges have not been established for the new site and are therefore not available, they can simply inform Dr. Patella that they cannot process the request until the privileges are offered at the new location.

New Technology, Equipment, and Procedures

A common challenge organizations face is failing to have a thorough process and well-written policy for implementing new technologies and medical techniques. Whenever an organization purchases new equipment or decides to offer a new medical technique, it not only must consider space, staffing, and resources, but it also must identify competence requirements needed for practitioners who will be using the equipment or the new technique if the technique is not simply an extension of their existing privileges. The credentials committee and the medical executive committee (MEC) should recommend and make revisions to competence requirements, and the governing body should base its decisions on those recommendations.

If a practitioner submits a request to perform a new procedure or a request to purchase and/or utilize new equipment and technology in which minimum threshold criteria have yet to be determined, your organization must first inform the applicant that the procedure is not available at this time. Your organization can review the procedure and determine whether it is a service that it wishes to offer. If the hospital determines that the procedure or new equipment is something it would like to pursue, the hospital can then follow the steps for developing and implementing the minimum threshold criteria outlined in Chapter 1.

The organization should also put the burden on the practitioner who has submitted the request to provide information about the new equipment or procedure, such as the following:

- Peer-reviewed research demonstrating the risks and benefits of the new equipment or procedure

- Product literature to support the proposed competence requirements

- Lists of other organizations that use the equipment or have implemented the procedure

- Vendor information and training information

If the organization determines that the new technology or equipment is not something that it supports at this time, then that feedback should be provided back to the practitioner who initially submitted the request.

If the medical staff and governing body determine that they do want to consider offering the new privileges, then the medical staff services department should follow the steps outlined in Chapter 1 for establishing minimum threshold criteria.

The MEC, department chair, and governing body should consider the following when deciding whether to offer a new procedure or technology, and these steps should be clearly outlined in a policy. In the example of Dr. Patella described at the beginning of the chapter, before the hospital can offer spine privileges at the new facility, the following would need to be considered and clearly outlined in the hospital's policy:

- **Resources:** What resources (space, funding, etc.) are required to support the new privileges/technology?

- **Equipment:** Is additional equipment required? If so, your organization must consider cost, maintenance, orientation and training, overhead, and cost-effectiveness. Additionally, the organization may want to determine whether the return on investment is worth the cost of the equipment.

- **Personnel:** Is there sufficient qualified staff to support the privileges being delineated? Will staff members need to be hired, trained, or otherwise affected?

- **Implementation:** What is a reasonable time frame to roll out the new privileges/technology? Are there any potential barriers that may need to be taken into consideration, and how will those be addressed?

The department chair, MEC, and the governing board need to consider each of these elements when evaluating requests for new privileges or technology. An organization also needs to revise the privilege delineations for the location(s) (if applicable) that this new procedure/technology would be offered if indeed it is determined that the request is a new privilege and not just an extension of a practitioner's existing privileges. Typically, if a procedure requires utilizing a new piece of equipment, additional education or training, is of a higher risk, or is not a transferable clinical skill, then it is more than just an extension of the practitioner's existing privileges. For example, if the new privileges are going to be offered at only two of four locations (in a multisystem organization), the privilege delineation would need to clearly reflect which two locations the new privileges can be carried out.

Once the MEC makes a recommendation and the governing body approves the criteria, interested practitioners have the opportunity to submit a request for the privileges along with documentation of current clinical competence that meets the minimum threshold criteria. If the organization determines that it does not want to offer the procedure, your organization should notify the applicant of its decision not to consider the request at this time. If the organization in the initial example approved offering spine privileges at the new location, Dr. Patella would then be able to resubmit his request for the new privilege at the new location.

Figures 10.1 and 10.2 provide sample algorithms that can be used to determine whether your organization should develop new privileging criteria for a new procedure or technology.

FIGURE 10.1

ALGORITHM FOR DECIDING WHEN TO DEVELOP CRITERIA

Procedure or therapy:

	Yes	No
1. Is the procedure within the scope of the hospital's plan of care?	Continue	Stop
2. Is the procedure of proven clinical efficacy and effectiveness and is it widely used in similar hospitals?	Continue	Consider whether or not the procedure will be permitted at all
3. Have at least two department chiefs agreed that the criteria needs to be developed?	Go to step 9	Continue
4. Is it likely that multiple specialties will be/are interested in this procedure?	Go to step 9	Continue
5. Have other organizations developed specific criteria for this procedure?	Go to step 9	Continue
6. Does the procedure represent a direct extension of existing clinical skills or judgment?	Consider adding the procedure to an existing block of core privileges	Continue
7. Does the procedure carry a risk greater than existing conventional therapy?	Go to step 9	Continue
8. Is the procedure of very recent introduction in your hospital or nationally?	Go to step 9	Consider adding the issue to an existing block of core practice privileging
9. Criteria should be developed. Proceed with procedure in form #3.		

 The Medical Staff's Guide to Overcoming Competence Assessment Challenges

FIGURE 10.1

ALGORITHM FOR DECIDING WHEN TO DEVELOP CRITERIA (CONT.)

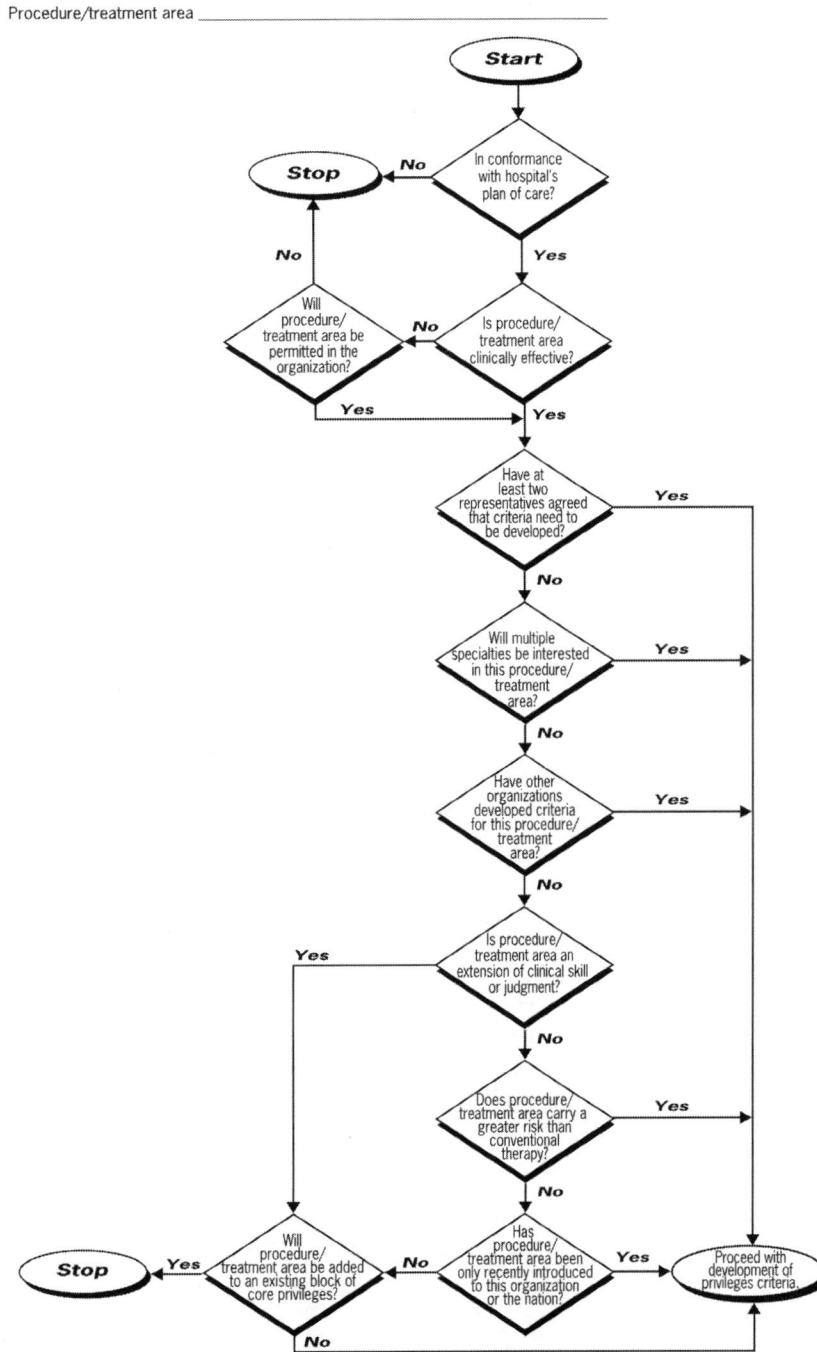

Procedure/treatment area _____

```
                              ( Start )
                                  │
                                  ▼
            No          ┌─────────────────┐
( Stop ) ◄──────────────┤  In conformance  │
                        │  with hospital's │
                        │  plan of care?   │
                        └─────────────────┘
    ▲                            │ Yes
    │ No                         ▼
┌──────────────┐      No  ┌─────────────────┐
│    Will      │◄─────────┤  Is procedure/  │
│  procedure/  │          │  treatment area │
│ treatment    │          │ clinically      │
│ area be      │          │ effective?      │
│ permitted in │          └─────────────────┘
│ the          │                   │ Yes
│ organization?│                   │
└──────────────┘                   │
      │ Yes                        ▼
      └──────────────►  ┌─────────────────┐
                        │    Have at       │      Yes
                        │   least two      ├────────────►
                        │ representatives  │
                        │ agreed that      │
                        │ criteria need to │
                        │ be developed?    │
                        └─────────────────┘
                                 │ No
                                 ▼
                        ┌─────────────────┐
                        │  Will multiple   │      Yes
                        │  specialties be  ├────────────►
                        │  interested in   │
                        │  this procedure/ │
                        │  treatment area? │
                        └─────────────────┘
                                 │ No
                                 ▼
                        ┌─────────────────┐
                        │  Have other      │      Yes
                        │  organizations   ├────────────►
                        │  developed       │
                        │  criteria for    │
                        │  this procedure/ │
                        │  treatment area? │
                        └─────────────────┘
                                 │ No
                                 ▼
                        ┌─────────────────┐
            Yes         │  Is procedure/   │
     ◄──────────────────┤  treatment area  │
                        │  an extension of │
                        │  clinical skill  │
                        │  or judgment?    │
                        └─────────────────┘
                                 │ No
                                 ▼
                        ┌─────────────────┐
                        │  Does procedure/ │      Yes
                        │  treatment area  ├────────────►
                        │  carry a greater │
                        │  risk than       │
                        │  conventional    │
                        │  therapy?        │
                        └─────────────────┘
                                 │ No
                                 ▼
┌─────────────┐   No    ┌─────────────────┐   Yes   ┌──────────────┐
│   Will      │◄────────┤  Has procedure/  ├────────►│  Proceed with │
│ procedure/  │         │  treatment area  │         │ development   │
│ treatment   │         │  been only       │         │ of privileges │
│ area be     │         │  recently        │         │ criteria.     │
│ added to an │         │  introduced to   │         └──────────────┘
│ existing    │         │  this            │
│ block of    │         │  organization or │
│ core        │         │  the nation?     │
│ privileges? │         └─────────────────┘
└─────────────┘
   │  │ Yes
   │No └──────────► ( Stop )
   │
   └─────────────────────────────────────────────────────►
```

FIGURE 10.2

ALGORITHM FOR PROCESS PRIVILEGING REQUESTS

Decision points	Yes	No
1. Is the request for an activity within the hospital's capability and has the hospital decided to provide such service?	Continue	Go to 8
2. Is the request for a contracted service?	Go to 5	Continue
3. Is the request for an item automatically granted to all physicians on the staff?	Go to 9	Continue
4. Are there criteria for determining if the request is valid?	Continue	Go to 7
5. Does the file document conformance to these criteria?	Go to 9	Go to 8
6. Has the director of contracted service indicated that the individual requesting privilege is an employee or independent contractor of the group?	Go to 3	Go to 8
7. Table the request and develop the criteria using current credentials Committee procedure (form #3). When complete, go to 4.		
8. Notify the applicant that the request will not be processed.		
9. Refer to department chief and credentials committee for review and recommendation (follow Credentials Committee procedure).		

 The Medical Staff's Guide to Overcoming Competence Assessment Challenges

FIGURE 10.2
ALGORITHM FOR PROCESS PRIVILEGING REQUESTS (CONT.)

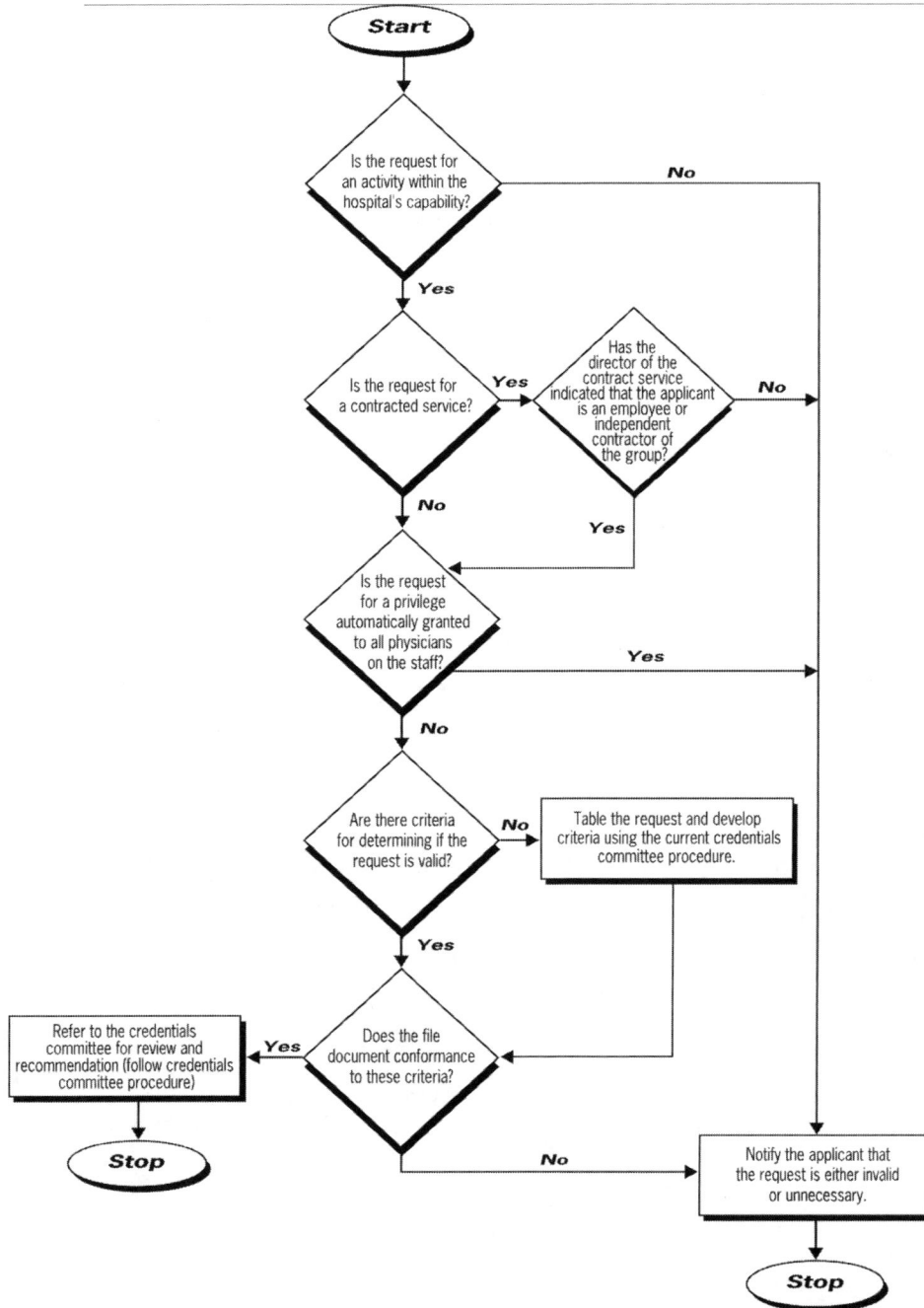

New Techniques

Often, practitioners want to perform a procedure in which the privileges are already developed; however, there is a new technique available to perform that procedure. Whenever a new technique is introduced, the organization must treat it as it would a request for a new procedure. It must also determine whether the new technique is of proven clinical efficacy and efficiency by evaluating the request as described throughout this chapter.

If the organization determines that the request is not an extension of a practitioner's existing skills and chooses to approve the new technique, then minimum threshold criteria for establishing current clinical competence must be developed as outlined in Chapter 1.

Additionally, whenever a new technique is approved, organizations should identify whether the new technique will require ancillary staff as well as the practitioner to undergo additional competence training. The medical staff services department must decide what experience it should require of the practitioners involved and how many cases should be proctored (please see Chapter 3 for a full explanation of proctoring).

Just as with requests for new technology or procedures, whenever a practitioner proposes a new technique, the organization should put the burden on the practitioner to provide the information needed for the credentials committee to conduct a thorough review and make an informed recommendation. The credentials committee has the responsibility of confirming all the information the practitioner provides, as well as gathering any additional information needed to conduct its assessment.

If the governing body approves the new technique, the organization should assess which privilege delineations need to be revised, at which locations the new technique would be performed, and what level of communication needs to occur as part of the implementation. For example, if multiple specialties will now use the new technique, each specialty would need to revise its privilege delineation form.

When reviewing requests for new privileges, techniques, and technology, organizations should also do the following, and this process should be clearly outlined in a policy:

- Invite all interested parties to provide input (interested parties will vary depending on request).

- Consider whether there are any exclusive contracts that may affect the option to offer the new privilege and whether the new privilege will be restricted to only practitioners covered under the exclusive contract.

- In addition to information the interested party provides, the organization must do its own research to ensure the medical staff and governing body have sufficient information to make an informed decision.

- Determine whether a technique is a new technique or just an extension of existing skills.

- Consider forming a new technology committee if there are a significant number of requests or if the medical staff sees value in appointing a committee to review these requests in detail.

- Ensure your organization has a knowledgeable and supportive culture to prevent practitioners from scheduling procedures that they do not have the appropriate privileges to perform. This can be achieved by educating the scheduling staff to verify that practitioners have the appropriate privileges prior to scheduling cases. Failure to educate your scheduling staff on verifying a practitioner's current privileges prior to scheduling can cause cases to be canceled or an organization to have to rush to process temporary privileges if there is a patient care need.

In summary, having a process and policy in place to evaluate requests for new techniques and equipment will ensure that your organization is prepared to respond to requests in a timely manner and take the necessary steps to develop the criteria if needed.

11

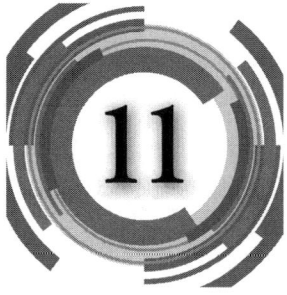

Low- and No-Volume Practitioners

Sally Pelletier, CPMSM, CPCS

CASE STUDY

The chief medical officer (CMO) of Midtown Memorial, a nonprofit, stand-alone healthcare system in a medium-size community, prepares for her weekly meeting with the director of medical staff services. In addition to reviewing the agenda for the upcoming credentials committee meeting, topics for discussion include the need to plan for the upcoming acquisition of Community General, a competing hospital, and its medical staff. The acquisition also includes the competing hospital's affiliated ambulatory clinics. It is anticipated that at least 20 new family medicine and internal medicine physicians, as well as a handful of subspecialties that include dermatology, allergy, and infectious disease, will be applying for staff membership and privileges. Most of these primary care practitioners, who will now become employees, will practice only in the office or clinic setting. The subspecialties will likely practice occasionally within the hospital as well as the clinic setting.

Although the CMO is new to her role, she trusts that the director of medical staff services is informed regarding this acquisition due to his participation in the development of a medical staff development plan, which is part of Midtown Memorial's governing body strategic planning process. Sure enough, the director of medical staff services, Mr. Meticulous, is not only aware of the acquisition, but he is also hoping that the acquisition will be the impetus for a needed revision to the medical staff bylaws, as well as a redesign of the organization's privileging forms.

Since the introduction of hospitalists at Midtown Memorial approximately five years ago, the director has voiced concerns to the chief of staff and the credentials committee chair that the medical staff bylaws are not conducive to the way practitioners currently practice medicine at Midtown.

In part, those concerns stem from the fact that the bylaws precisely link membership on the medical staff with clinical privileges and that a physician must have an active hospital practice with at least 20 annual admissions to be eligible for membership on the medical staff. Mr. Meticulous repeats those concerns at every reappointment cycle when the family medicine and internal medicine physicians who increasingly choose to utilize the hospitalists continue to request active staff membership and inpatient privileges. The internal and family medicine physicians refer patients to hospitalists so frequently that their clinical activity level in the hospital setting is minimal to nonexistent.

The CMO and the director decide that it is past time to deal with the necessary bylaw revisions and make note of the necessity to convene the bylaws committee as an action item. The CMO offers to contact the bylaws committee chair and to ask that he assemble the committee with the following goals in mind:

- The medical staff (and subsequently, the governing board) will separate decisions related to privileges from decisions related to medical staff membership

- Appointment of a practitioner to a specific medical staff membership category will support the medical staff's desire to enfranchise practitioners who fulfill an important strategic role and support the mission of the medical staff and the hospital

- Medical staff categories will be revisited and revised as appropriate to reflect the changes in practice that have transpired at Midtown over the course of the past several years

Mr. Meticulous agrees with the goals as stated and provides the CMO with additional insight as to why the bylaws need to be revised, including the fact that they:

- Inhibit or prevent effective processing of medical staff membership requests made by low- and no-volume practitioners by requiring that practitioners on the active medical staff perform a certain number of procedures at the facility.

- Require physicians to receive referrals from the emergency department (ED) or participate in medical staff affairs.

- State that a physician must be on the active staff at another facility for the hospital to grant him or her courtesy appointment. (This requirement was designed to ensure that all physicians are subject to at least one medical staff's peer review process and that they are required to fulfill medical staff responsibilities.)

- Require initial appointment to a provisional category to allow the medical staff to observe an applicant's initial work before deciding whether to appoint him or her to the active or courtesy staff category. (This category has now typically been supplanted by the Joint Commission requirement to implement a period of focused professional practice evaluation [FPPE] for all initial requests for privileges.)

The CMO and the director turn their attention to the credentials committee agenda. The director begins to review the reappointment applications of concern that are to be presented at the credentials committee meeting. Those files include Dr. Cosmo, who is a dermatologist; Dr. Cares-A-Lot, who is a family medicine practitioner; and Dr. Sneezer, who is an allergist. The director points out that for each of these physicians, the feedback reports that display clinical activity and the results of their periodic appraisal and performance monitoring contain little to no information. He also points out that Dr. Cosmo and Dr. Sneezer are not on the active staff, so they are not subject to the requirement for 20 admissions. He explains to the CMO that he is hesitant to present these files to the department of medicine chair for review because he and his department have been unable to obtain evidence of current proficiency related to clinical privileges granted.

Introduction to Low- and No-Volume Practitioners

Changes occurring in hospitals and medical staff practices today increasingly challenge hospitals with how best to address practitioners who have little or no clinical care volume in the hospital (hereinafter referred to as low-volume and no-volume practitioners). The forces driving these changes are powerful and growing, including:

- Rapid growth of hospitalist programs

- Outpatient settings offering better practitioner productivity with fewer hassles

- Physicians seeking enhanced revenues from provider-owned outpatient facilities

- Technological advances expanding the minimally invasive procedures that can safely be performed in outpatient settings

- Increasing numbers of practitioners seeking a better balance for their professional and personal lives

- Practitioners' active efforts to reduce or avoid ED call responsibilities

These forces are creating an ever-growing number of practitioners who practice in the community yet have little or no practice at the hospital. Some of these practitioners still want to maintain a relationship with the hospital and its medical staff, while others do not. Sometimes a practitioner's interest in clinical privileges is driven solely by insurance companies' and managed care plans' requirement that practitioners on their panels maintain hospital privileges. Yet even this requirement is going by the wayside in a growing number of markets.

The approach your organization takes to gathering evidence of a low- or no-volume practitioner's competence depends on the reason(s) for which the practitioner sees few patients or performs few to no clinical procedures at your organization. We will use this chapter to explore specific approaches based on the type of low- or no-volume practitioner. We have already learned in Chapter 9 how to assess the single practitioner in a specialty area. Chapter 12 will address practitioners who selectively practice, making it difficult to determine their competence for the full core privileges and call coverage. Therefore, this chapter will primarily deal with those practitioners who are not clinically active at your hospital:

- But are active at another hospital

- But are active at an ambulatory clinic and do not have a relationship with the hospital

- But are primarily office-based; this will be addressed from both an employed and nonemployed perspective

By now, healthcare organizations and those individuals involved in the credentialing and privileging process must realize that regulatory bodies are placing greater emphasis on linking privileges with demonstrated current competence. At the same time, the increasing number of non-hospital-based practitioners creates a challenge for maintaining effective and productive relationships between these practitioners and the hospital to support the hospital's mission, vision, and strategic plan.

Together, the greater emphasis on linking privileges with competence and an increasing number of hospital-based practitioners make it critical for hospitals to achieve the following three goals:

  The Medical Staff's Guide to Overcoming Competence Assessment Challenges

- Meet legal and regulatory requirements

- Ensure all practitioners are granted only privileges for which they have demonstrated current competence

- Build and maintain strategic relationships between the hospital and practitioners who rarely or never practice within the organization

Assessing the Competence of the Practitioner Who Is Active at Another Facility

Let us first address the practitioner who is clinically active at another facility with very little or no activity in your organization. Medical services professionals (MSP) see these types of cases all the time when they credential a new practitioner's request for clinical privileges when that practitioner has been actively practicing elsewhere. Thus, MSPs should be very familiar with the tools and techniques that allow them to gather evidence of current competence. Those tools and techniques include the following (remember, put the burden on the applicant to obtain the required information):

1. If the low- or no-volume practitioner has significant clinical activity at another facility that is reflective of the scope of clinical privileges that he or she is requesting at your facility, send a peer reference questionnaire to responsible individuals at that site (e.g., department chair, section chief) seeking confirmation of the practitioner's medical/clinical knowledge, technical and clinical skills, clinical judgment, interpersonal skills, professionalism, absence of disciplinary issues, judgment, behavior, and any additional factors relevant to making recommendations for clinical privileges.

2. In addition, seek references from those individuals who can attest to the practitioner's interpersonal skills, professionalism, absence of disciplinary issues, judgment, and behavior (e.g., hospital's CEO, director of medical records, directors of clinical units).

3. Collect volume data as available from the ongoing professional practice evaluation (OPPE) from the other institution. To gather this information, put the burden on the practitioner applying for privileges. The practitioner should ensure the provision of all elements that are required by your organization, including:

- Process data

    - Nationally required core measures (physician relevant)

    - Blood use data

    - Illegibility/nonapproved-abbreviation incidents

    - Patient complaints

- Outcomes data

    - Claims-based data (e.g., C-sections, complications, mortality rates [preferably risk adjusted])

    - State public databases

    - Peer review final case ratings

- Volume of clinical activity at the other facility for the past six to 12 months

    - Admissions

    - Procedures

    - Deliveries

- Confirmation of medical staff status "in good standing" with no disciplinary actions, no contemplated investigations, and no ongoing investigations or quality/peer review adverse actions

Let's revisit our case study.

Dr. Rose and Dr. Cares-A-Lot: Two Solutions to the Low- and No-Volume Challenge

Fortunately, the new CMO and the seasoned director of the medical staff services from Midtown Memorial recognize the strategic importance of separating membership from clinical privileges. They know that many hospitals and medical staffs have medical staff categories that allow practitioners to maintain a relationship with the hospital without clinical privileges. This collegial solution to what is a very common problem requires careful and thoughtful design of membership categories and should be done with the end goal or goals in mind. Those goals will be specific to each organization but will likely include:

- Building and maintaining strategic relationships between the hospital and independent practitioners who rarely or never practice within the organization

- The granting of privileges based on the degree to which the practitioner meets the criteria for privileges requested, including evidence of current competence

- Adopting a simpler, more rational approach to medical staff categories

The CMO works with Mr. Meticulous and the bylaws committee chair to convene a series of bylaws committee meetings. The committee needs some education about this concept of separating membership from privileges and asks Mr. Meticulous to prepare a presentation to the committee. The presentation and discussion center on the following concepts:

- The term credentialing refers to the overall process of gathering and verifying credentials information, reviewing that information, and making a decision to grant or deny medical staff membership. Although appointing physicians to the medical staff and granting clinical privileges are part of the credentialing process, they are not one and the same.

- Medical staff membership most commonly involves the creation of specific categories that address voting rights and whether a physician is allowed to hold office. In addition, depending on the organization's policies, membership allows physicians access to the physicians' dining room, hospital library, continuing medical education (CME) classes, and other benefits befitting membership. In addition, granting membership allows physicians to advertise their affiliation with the organization and satisfy managed care organizations' requirements, if applicable.

- Physicians who seek only medical staff appointment should complete an application or reapplication form, submit letters or completed reference questionnaires from colleagues, and provide a description of their private practices or practices at another facility.

- Appointing a physician to the medical staff does not automatically allow him or her to treat patients. Therefore, Midtown's credentials committee can recommend medical staff membership for a low- or no-volume practitioner who desires to be affiliated with Midtown but who does not want or need privileges to admit and treat patients.

Mr. Meticulous also points out that Midtown's current membership criteria require members to provide ED on-call coverage and specifically state that all members must hold clinical privileges. This is the reason the organization does not currently have the option of appointing a physician to the medical staff without also granting privileges. He concludes by stating that contemporary bylaws separate membership from privileges and allow for physicians to join an appropriate staff category with or without clinical privileges. The bylaws should also detail the responsibilities of practitioners appointed to these staff categories.

Ultimately, the bylaws committee works hard and, over the course of several meetings, ends up with several recommendations that are later adopted by the organized medical staff and the hospital's governing body, resulting in a contemporary set of medical staff bylaws.

Addressing the separation of membership from clinical privileges and adopting a more rational approach to medical staff categories via a revision to the medical staff bylaws will provide an option for Midtown to address the referring physicians who are practicing independently and are not clinically active in the hospital or hospital-affiliated entities but continue to request reappointment to the medical staff. The following story about Dr. Rose, who has previously held active family medicine privileges at Midtown, may make it easier to understand the application of such an option.

Frank Rose, MD, is a family physician who has been a member of Midtown Memorial's medical staff for 15 years. Dr. Rose practices as an independent private practitioner and has an active office-based ambulatory practice. Over the past 15 years, Dr. Rose has routinely admitted and cared for patients at Midtown when they were in need of inpatient services. However, due to a desire to achieve a better work–life balance and to escape some of the bureaucracy of the hospital setting, Dr. Rose has decided to concentrate his medical practice on treating patients solely in his office setting.

As a result of this decision, Dr. Rose made arrangements with the hospitalist group at Midtown to provide inpatient care to his patients. This arrangement, now in its second year, is working well for Dr. Rose, his patients, the hospitalists, and the hospital. However, because of the efficiency and reliability of the hospitalists, Dr. Rose has not provided clinical services to hospital patients in more than one year. Despite the absence of clinical inpatient work, Dr. Rose remains active in the hospital's family medicine department and regularly attends hospital-sponsored CME.

Dr. Rose was recently up for reappointment. In accordance with the hospital's bylaws, he submitted a reapplication form to the medical staff services department. His completed reapplication includes a request for "continued privileges in family medicine."

The medical staff bylaws state that the organization will evaluate privilege requests based on competence data gathered through the hospital's performance improvement program. This requirement hinders Dr. Rose's renewal of family medicine privileges because he does not provide inpatient services at Midtown or any other hospital. The department chair does not have access to data that can attest to his current clinical competence in this area. The chair is therefore concerned that he will be forced to deny Dr. Rose's request for privileges.

The department chair then recalls that the recent discussion among the medical staff members that led to the bylaws revision provided a new category of membership, known as the "affiliate" category. This category is reserved for members who maintain a clinical practice in the hospital service area and wish to be able to follow the course of their patients when admitted to the hospital—exactly the scenario in which Dr. Rose finds himself. Although Dr. Rose is no longer eligible for clinical privileges and would not be able to manage patient care in the hospital, vote on medical staff affairs, or hold office, as a member of the affiliate category, he would be allowed to order noninvasive outpatient diagnostic tests and services, visit patients in the hospital, review medical records, and attend medical staff meetings, CME functions, and social events. Because physicians like Dr. Rose are not fully exercising hospital inpatient privileges anyway, most are happy to accept this type of approach, maintain medical staff membership, and continue to serve on committees, use the library, and attend medical staff meetings.

> **TIP**
>
> Before processing the physician's request for privileges, hospital and medical staff leaders should engage in a collegial conversation with the physician applicant to determine whether he or she is interested in privileges that authorize him or her to treat patients on an inpatient basis. This discussion should include providing the practitioner with information regarding their clinical activity (volume and scope) at your organization.

The department chair resolves that Dr. Rose may be reappointed to the affiliate category. He plans to have a conversation with Dr. Rose to inform him that he is no longer eligible to request inpatient privileges in family medicine, believing that this approach is a strategic "win-win" for both parties. Dr. Rose already supports the hospital's mission by directing all his patients to the institution's hospitalist program or staff consultants for inpatient treatment, sending all his patients in need of emergency care to the hospital, and relying on the facility's outpatient services for tests and therapy (e.g., radiology, physical therapy, and occupational therapy). For all these reasons, the department chair recognizes the value this type of physician has in his or her relationship with the hospital, and he is thankful that they finally have the right kind of solution in place for Dr. Rose. He is also thankful that his workload will be reduced, because when processing applications submitted by physicians who simply refer patients to the hospital for treatment, the organization does not have to determine their competence, because they are not treating patients.

If an organization decides to grant a physician membership without privileges, it is not obligated to confirm the physician's clinical competence, because the practitioner does not seek to exercise privileges at the organization. All of his or her patients in need of acute hospital services would receive those services through direct referral by this physician to other medical staff members with clinical privileges. Mr. Meticulous makes a note of this in Memorial's credentialing policies and procedures. During the next reappointment cycle, Mr. Meticulous and the staff in the medical staff services department gather information demonstrating Dr. Rose's compliance with basic appointment criteria established by the medical staff bylaws, including two letters from Dr. Rose's colleagues that confirm that he is in good standing in the medical community. This information allows the credentials committee to determine that Dr. Rose's continued medical staff appointment would not jeopardize the hospital's or medical staff's reputation in the community.

The department chair then turns his attention to the next credentials file, Dr. Cares-A-Lot, the family medicine physician who is applying for initial appointment as a result of the acquisition of Community General. At first glance, the department chair wonders if Dr. Cares-A-Lot would fit into the affiliate category. He then recalls a recent conversation with Mr. Meticulous regarding the Joint Commission's requirement to privilege practitioners (employed and non-employed) who practice in the ambulatory settings that undergo the same survey process as the hospital (essentially, the ambulatory setting is a department of the hospital). He realizes that the affiliate category would not be the right fit for Dr. Cares-A-Lot and begins to review the privilege delineation form included with the application that is specific to the ambulatory clinic setting.

Dr. Cares-A-Lot and Dr. Rose are examples of one of the fastest growing trends in medicine today: the primary care physician who no longer practices in the hospital. The medical staff and the hospital administration at Midtown had already discussed what kind of relationship they wanted to have with this new group of low- and no-volume practitioners. During the previous discussion of the bylaws committee recommendations, the medical staff and the hospital administration decided that a relationship with this group of primary care physicians is important for the membership of the medical staff despite their lack of inpatient care. This was one reason for the decision they made to separate membership criteria from privileging criteria. Additionally, Midtown needed to create ambulatory privileges for practitioners who are not currently competent to provide inpatient care and should not request inpatient privileges.

Matching Privileges to Current Competence

This leads us to a discussion regarding the medical staff's responsibility to match privileges with current competence—one of the biggest challenges that low- and no-volume practitioners present. Public awareness, demand for high-quality healthcare, and stringent requirements from accrediting and regulatory bodies regarding practitioner competence put increasing pressure on healthcare organizations to match privileges with current clinical competence. The Joint Commission refers to an "assessment of current competence to perform requested privileges" as a proviso for granting clinical privileges. The Joint Commission defines competence or competency as "a determination of an individual's skills, knowledge, and capability to meet defined expectations." Although The Joint Commission does not specifically define "current," we can make some reasonable assumptions.

TIP

Answering the competency equation is an effective means of procuring the information your service chief, department chair, credentials committee, and medical executive committee (MEC) need prior to making a recommendation regarding clinical privileges. The competency equation is simply:

Competency = Have you done it recently? + When you did it, did you do it well?

To fulfill the competence equation, the medical staff services department must gather evidence of performance directly related to the practitioner's request for clinical privileges. In addition, it must gather data related to the quality (outcomes) of the procedures or privileges performed.

Some practitioners argue that performing certain procedures is like riding a bicycle, and whether they performed a certain procedure recently is immaterial. Certainly, the clinical skills required to maintain proficiency for various procedures may vary depending on the complexity of the procedure. However, if we think outside of a clinical context, all of us can identify jobs, tasks, or hobbies for which we may have been well qualified in the past but would require practice and preparation to achieve the same level of proficiency today.

Some practitioners also argue that the volume of procedures performed is not a good indicator of competence. It is important to note that neither function of the competence equation is sufficient on its own. The number of times a practitioner performs a privilege or procedure is not sufficient if it is not accompanied by data regarding the quality of the practitioner's performance.

Likewise, practitioner performance profiles, professional reference questionnaires, and statements submitted by the practitioner's service chief or department chair do not provide complete information about competence if the practitioner has not engaged in a clinical activity recently.

In theory, organizations that struggle to gather adequate clinical data for low- and no-volume practitioners fail to establish the link between privileges and competence because they have not updated their delineation of privileges to accurately define the care, treatment, and services provided by their practitioners or they have not defined correlating performance measures.

As mentioned earlier in this chapter and throughout this book, matching the clinical privileges a practitioner requests to his or her demonstrated current competence is critical. To accomplish this goal, hospitals need to develop and maintain a criteria-based privileging system that accurately defines the services currently offered by the facility and appropriately reflects the scope of services provided by each of its practitioners.

Criterion-based privileging systems establish predefined qualifications, such as education, training, previous experience, and demonstrated current competence, that an applicant or reapplicant must meet to request specific procedures or privileges.

In summary, privileging systems should be designed to ensure that every practitioner has been approved to hold certain privileges based on an evaluation of his or her licensure, training, experience, and current competence. Privileges should be criteria-based, meaning that the organization should establish minimal qualifications that a practitioner must meet to be eligible to apply for specific privileges. The organization must assess and reassess each practitioner using the competence equation before granting or regranting privileges.

The following concepts are the guiding principles for addressing low- and no-volume practitioners. The Donabedian Triangle, which ties together structure, process, and outcomes, provides the framework for The Greeley Company's competency triangle. (Figure 11.1)

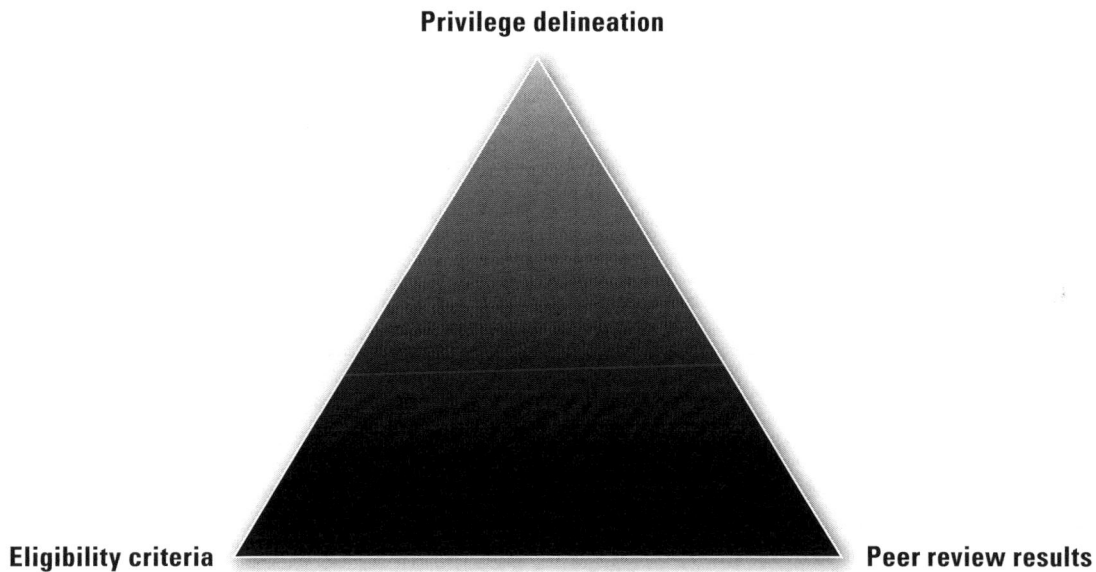

FIGURE 11.1

THE GREELEY COMPETENCY TRIANGLE

The Competency Triangle

Privilege delineation

Eligibility criteria

Peer review results

Each corner of the triangle is key to creating an effective competence management system. If a negative outcome occurs, an evaluation of the process and structure is warranted to determine whether either one falls short. For example, if a family medicine practitioner experiences negative outcomes related to deliveries, a review of the eligibility criteria may provide credentialing professionals insight as to whether the criteria are appropriate or need to be revised.

In the case of Dr. Cares-A-Lot and the other primary care practitioners who were previously affiliated with Community General, the plan is for them to continue to provide primary care in offices that operate under the license of the hospital. Unlike independent offices for which the hospital has no obligations (as was the case with Dr. Rose), the hospital will be required to have a process in place for evaluating the competence of the physicians (employed or not) practicing in these offices. This does not necessarily mean that the physicians have to become members of the medical staff, but the hospital must have a process to determine the competence of the physicians in their outpatient practices. In the same way that inpatient data and measurement is defined, collected, reviewed, and acted on, the outpatient data the medical staff services department gathers must also prove the physician's current competence in an ambulatory setting.

In contrast to the primary care physicians whose inpatient clinical privileges do not correspond with care they are providing in the ambulatory setting, certain specialties (e.g., dermatologists, allergists, infectious disease specialists) may very well be providing the same type of care in the hospital setting at Midtown as they are providing in the office setting. Accordingly, their privileges need to accurately depict the care, treatment, and services they are performing in both settings, and then their proficiency for those privileges must be confirmed through established or appropriately developed medical staff mechanisms.

It is important to note that if a practitioner wishes to maintain clinical privileges that allow him or her to actively treat acutely ill patients, he or she must provide evidence that demonstrates current clinical competence. In short, he or she must ensure that the competency equation is met to the satisfaction of the department chair and credentials committee. However, the practitioner in question may have difficulty providing this information because he or she has not recently provided care to acutely ill patients and is therefore unable to demonstrate inpatient performance results. Some credentials committees would have significant difficulty if faced with this dilemma.

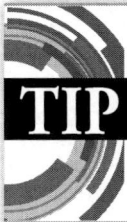

TIP

When a practitioner seeks clinical privileges for authorization to treat acutely ill patients but cannot provide evidence demonstrating the skills necessary to provide such treatment, it is not the credentials committee's responsibility to prove that the physician is competent. It is the practitioner's responsibility to furnish evidence demonstrating that he or she meets the minimum threshold criteria established by the medical staff for clinical privileges requested.

Avoid Denying Privileges

When it becomes apparent that there is a need to modify requests for clinical privileges, there are options available to credentials committees other than denying privileges. Credentials committees are permitted, when necessary, to request that a practitioner modify his or her request for clinical privileges. This option is particularly important when there is a chance that the practitioner's privileging request may be formally denied.

Department chairs should not hesitate to alert the credentials committee and MEC when they are unable to assess current clinical competence due to the absence of information. The credentials committee or MEC must then use its experience, skills, and knowledge to appropriately respond to this unusual circumstance. By the time a request reaches the credentials committee or MEC, the department chair and medical staff services department have determined whether the practitioner meets established criteria for membership and/ or clinical privileges.

Most experienced credentialing professionals recognize the importance of avoiding denials, and therefore avoiding potential reporting to the National Practitioner Data Bank or state licensing bodies, and use other techniques, such as establishing clear membership and privileging criteria, to ensure that quality patient care is delivered in a safe environment. With clear criteria in place, organizations are unable to process an applicant's file if they fail to meet established criteria. The following guidelines are worth repeating and should help credentials committees respond to medical staff membership and privileging requests made by low- and no-volume practitioners:

- Unfortunately, as previously mentioned, many medical staffs have not permitted their bylaws to evolve to adequately handle these new circumstances. A review of your organization's bylaws will reveal whether they offer the proper guidance or need to be revised and updated to address today's credentialing and privileging challenges.

- Credentials committees often overanalyze such situations to avoid insulting or criticizing a colleague. However, the best course of action is to deal with any circumstance that might result in a denial of privileges in a businesslike manner. Rely on your policies and procedures to avoid the appearance of impropriety.

- Communicate, communicate, communicate with the low- and no-volume practitioner regarding established criteria for clinical privileges, volumes incurred at your facility, intended practice plan status, the increased focus on determining proficiency for clinical privileges granted, and the strategic direction of your medical staff.

- Remember the overlying general principle that requires hospitals to grant privileges only after reviewing data that attest to a practitioner's current clinical competence specific to the privileges requested.

12

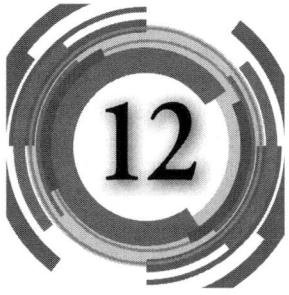

Selective Practice Affecting Competence, Privileges, and Call Coverage

Sally Pelletier, CPMSM, CPCS

CASE STUDY

At Specialized Medical Center, the CEO, chief medical officer (CMO), and the president of the medical staff are becoming increasingly alarmed at the number of physicians who are making significant modifications to their core privileges and then saying they are no longer able to cover the emergency department (ED) for their respective specialties. This is occurring more frequently with colorectal surgeons, breast surgeons, spine surgeons, orthopedic and plastic hand surgeons, and orthopedists who are limiting their practice to hip and knee replacements. As a result, the ED is developing a critical shortage of needed specialists to provide call coverage.

At one point, the CEO, CMO, and president of the medical staff thought that core privileging would ensure that every specialist had enough privileges to cover the ED. However, the director of medical staff services reminded them of the Center for Medicare & Medicaid Services' (CMS) and The Joint Commission's requirements that make it clear that physicians need to be able to modify or opt out of some portions of the core privileges if they did not wish to request them. CMS made this directive clear in its memo from November 2004 ("CMS Requirements for Hospital Medical Staff Privileging"). The Joint Commission clarified its position in a frequently asked question (FAQ) list from November 2008.

The hospital has to transfer more and more patients due to lack of available specialists. Administration is becoming concerned about vulnerability of a "dumping" complaint from another hospital under the Emergency Medical Treatment and Active Labor Act (EMTALA). It is equally concerned with the loss of patient revenues and a declining local reputation due to the hospital transferring patients for relatively basic services that it should be able to provide to the community.

Solution/Discussion

More and more hospitals are dealing with practitioners with limited activity because they choose to limit their practices and focus on becoming highly specialized. An orthopedist may limit his or her practice to hip and knee replacements. A general surgeon may choose to become a highly specialized breast surgeon. It is important in these scenarios to make sure the practitioners' clinical privileges are:

- Accurately delineated

- Recommended based on established criteria that take into account the physician's education, training, and current experience

- Granted based on evidence of current clinical competence

The problem facing many hospitals today is the challenge of managing ED call coverage issues. Problems surrounding ED call coverage come from a variety of different areas and have a variety of solutions. This chapter specifically addresses how these types of selective practices affect an organization's ability to determine competence for those practitioners who choose to limit their privileges. In certain cases, these same practitioners also insist that because they do not hold certain privileges, they cannot take ED call. Organizations must confirm the physician's competence for the full scope of privileges he or she requests. However, in these scenarios where the issue of covering call also muddies the waters, there may not be a clear understanding of what EMTALA requires.

WHAT IS CORE PRIVILEGING?

Core privileging is an effective criterion-based approach to privileging that uses predefined eligibility criteria in conjunction with a clinically realistic, well-defined description of "core" privileges for each specific clinical specialty or subspecialty treatment area. Core privileges are facility-specific and recognize procedures that would be considered within a practitioner's competencies based on the completion of an approved postgraduate training program. Recent confirmed experience combined with good outcomes form the basis for determining competence for both the core and those special or non-core procedures that may require additional training or competencies that are of a higher risk or introduce a new technology or technique.

 The Medical Staff's Guide to Overcoming Competence Assessment Challenges

This chapter is not dedicated to a discussion of all the intricacies that go into developing a workable solution to ED call coverage. However, it does suggest one simple step that, if implemented, helps to manage this conundrum as it relates to privileging—and even more specifically, to core privileging: add EMTALA language to privileging forms.

Add EMTALA-Based Language to Privileging Forms

Language that addresses the EMTALA requirements to assess, stabilize, and determine a patient's condition can be added to your delineation of privilege forms as applicable to each specialty for which the medical executive committee (MEC) has established call coverage requirements. The language can simply be stated as follows: "Assess, stabilize, and determine disposition of patients with emergent conditions consistent with medical staff policy regarding emergency and consultative call services."

For organizations that utilize the core privileging methodology, this statement should be included in the initial description of the core. Physicians who hold privileges in their respective specialty areas but may not qualify for the full set of core privileges should be competent to assess and stabilize the patient and then transfer care as appropriate. For example, an orthopedist who specializes in hips or knees is competent to assess a patient with a dislocated shoulder and make the determination as to where to transfer the care of the patient as appropriate.

For organizations that utilize laundry list privileges, the same language could be inserted as a matter of policy for any practitioners who are requesting privileges in their areas of practice in accordance with the MEC's established requirements for call coverage by specialty.

The problem of ED call coverage is not easily fixed and requires thoughtful discussion and negotiation between all parties involved (e.g., physicians, senior administration, and medical staff leadership). However, organizations can provide guidance and clarification within their privileging forms by adding language that addresses what is required by EMTALA, as noted above.

Call coverage aside, department chairs and credentials committees must use caution when evaluating and recommending privileges for, as an example, the orthopedist who chooses to focus on hip and knee replacements in his or her private practice but takes call for general orthopedics at the hospital. The competency equation discussed in Chapter 11 is still applicable.

The competency equation puts the burden on the applicant to prove not only that he or she has provided a service or procedure (volume) but also that he or she has done it well (outcomes). When your organization establishes volumes as one of the qualifications for privileges, it should require physicians to perform a minimum number of procedures—not a maximum—to maintain their skills. The push to link competence to clinical privileges is why it is so important to accurately delineate or describe the clinical privileges being requested and granted.

ED Call Coverage for Practitioners Who Are Not Competent to Assess, Stabilize, and Determine the Disposition of Patients

Practitioners covering ED call who have limited their practices should be held to criteria that require them to be able to assess, stabilize, and determine patient conditions. However, there may be some point where they are no longer proficient to handle even this minimal requirement. This will require continual assessment of the practitioner's skills for the core in his or her specialty area.

Most medical staff bylaws and/or rules and regulations require the medical staff member to fulfill an obligation to cover ED call, as appropriate for the specialty. In years past, assignment on the call roster was considered a benefit and a way to build the practitioner's patient load. Thus, medical staff bylaws allowed the "active" medical staff the opportunity to cover call. Conversely, "courtesy" staff could not cover call. In many organizations, covering ED call is no longer considered a benefit, and therefore a different approach is needed.

This change has led many organizations to rethink how they manage ED call. Many medical staffs have also determined that a one-size-fits-all approach for each medical staff category or clinical specialty is also not effective. A solution created by some organizations is to delegate the responsibility for creating requirements for call roster obligations to the medical staff departments and/or service lines, which will then reside in an MEC-approved policy. Thus, each clinical area recommends how call obligations will be defined (e.g., pediatrics, OB/GYN, general surgery, orthopedics, etc.) with MEC approval. This is an excellent practice.

Returning to the issue of the practitioner who can no longer demonstrate competence to assess, stabilize, and determine disposition of patients with emergent conditions, the obligation to serve call is still present. The burden is on the practitioner to provide alternative call coverage arrangements by getting someone else in his or her group or another practitioner within the same specialty to cover for him or her.

Some organizations are evolving in their privilege delineation methodology from core to clusters to address specialized areas of focus (e.g., general surgeons who are performing only breast surgery and orthopedists subspecializing in hips, knees, total joints, or sports medicine). The principle behind the creation of privileging clusters is the same as for core: that is, to create, through a narrative (and a back-up procedure list as applicable to the specialized area of focus), a description of what privileges are included in the cluster and the eligibility requirements for an applicant or a reapplicant to request the cluster. Figures 12.1 and 12.2 are two examples:

FIGURE 12.1
BREAST SURGERY CLUSTER – GENERAL SURGEONS

Qualifications:

EDUCATION: Successful completion of an Accreditation Council for Graduate Medical Education (ACGME)- or American Osteopathic Association (AOA)-accredited residency in general surgery.

AND/OR

BOARD CERTIFICATION: Current certification board eligibility leading to certification in general surgery by the American Board of Surgery or the American Osteopathic Board of Surgery.

AND

EXPERIENCE: At least 100 breast surgery procedures with acceptable results, reflective of the scope of privileges requested, during the past 12 months or demonstrate successful completion of an ACGME- or AOA-accredited residency or clinical fellowship within the past 12 months.

Reappointment (Renewal of Privileges) Requirements: To be eligible to renew privileges in breast surgery, the reapplicant must meet the following criteria:

Current demonstrated competence and an adequate volume of experience (200 breast surgery procedures) with acceptable results, reflective of the scope of privileges requested, for the past 24 months based on results of ongoing professional practice evaluation and outcomes.

Evidence of current physical and mental ability to perform privileges requested is required of all applicants for renewal of privileges.

FIGURE 12.1

BREAST SURGERY CLUSTER – GENERAL SURGEONS (CONT.)

PRIVILEGES – BREAST SURGERY

- Requested   Admit, evaluate, diagnose, consult with, provide pre-, intra-, and postoperative care to, and perform surgical procedures on patients of all ages, to correct or treat various conditions, diseases, disorders, and injuries of the breast. May provide care to patients in the intensive care setting in conformance with unit policies. Assess, stabilize, and determine disposition of patients with emergent conditions consistent with medical staff policy regarding emergency and consultative call services.

This list is a sampling of procedures included in the primary cluster. This is not intended to be an all-encompassing list but rather reflective of the categories/types of procedures included in the cluster.

To the applicant: If you wish to exclude any procedures, please strike through those procedures that you do not wish to request, initial, and date.

1. Perform history and physical exam
2. Complete mastectomy with or without axillary lymph node dissection
3. Excision of breast lesion
4. Breast biopsy
5. Incision and drainage of abscess
6. Modified radical mastectomy
7. Operation for gynecomastia
8. Partial mastectomy with or without lymph node dissection
9. Radical mastectomy
10. Subcutaneous mastectomy

(The following could be special procedures with additional training and experience required.)

1. Sentinel node biopsy
2. Stereotactic breast biopsy
3. Breast cryoablation

   The Medical Staff's Guide to Overcoming Competence Assessment Challenges

FIGURE 12.2

SURGERY OF THE HAND

Qualifications: To be eligible to apply for privileges in surgery of the hand, the initial applicant must meet the following criteria:

Education: Successful completion of an Accreditation Council for Graduate Medical Education (ACGME)–or American Osteopathic Association (AOA)–accredited residency in general, orthopedic, or plastic surgery and successful completion of an accredited fellowship in hand surgery.

AND/OR

Board Certification: Current subspecialty certification or board eligibility in surgery of the hand by the American Board of Surgery, the American Board of Orthopedic Surgery, or the American Board of Plastic Surgery; or Certificate of Added Qualifications in Hand Surgery by the American Osteopathic Board of Orthopedic Surgery.

AND

EXPERIENCE: At least 50 surgery-of-the-hand procedures, reflective of the scope of privileges requested, within the past 12 months, or successful completion of an ACGME- or AOA-accredited residency or clinical fellowship within the past 12 months.

Reappointment (Renewal of Privileges) Requirements: To be eligible to renew privileges in surgery of the hand, the reapplicant must meet the following criteria:

Current demonstrated competence and an adequate volume of experience (100 hand procedures) with acceptable results, reflective of the scope of privileges requested, for the past 24 months based on results of ongoing professional practice evaluation and outcomes.

Evidence of current physical and mental ability to perform privileges requested is required of all applicants for renewal of privileges.

CORE PRIVILEGES – SURGERY OF THE HAND

- Requested   Admit, evaluate, diagnose, treat, and provide consultation (includes investigation, preservation, and restoration) for patients of all ages by medical, surgical, and rehabilitative means of all structures of the upper extremity directly affecting the form and function of the hand and wrist. May provide care to patients in the intensive care setting in conformance with unit policies. Assess, stabilize, and determine disposition of patients with emergent conditions consistent with medical staff policy regarding emergency and consultative call services. The core privileges in this specialty include the following procedures and such other procedures that are extensions of the same techniques and skills. **To the applicant:** If you wish to exclude any procedures, please strike through those procedures that you do not wish to request, initial, and date.

- Perform history and physical exam

- Amputation (related to hand/upper extremity)

FIGURE 12.2
SURGERY OF THE HAND (CONT.)

- Arthroscopy

- Bone grafts and corrective osteotomies

- Dupuytren's contracture

- Fasciotomy, deep incision and drainage for infection, and wound debridement

- Foreign body and implant removal

- Joint and tendon sheath repairs, including release of contracture, synovectomy, arthroplasty with and without implant, arthrodesis, trigger finger release, and stiff joints that result from rheumatoid or other injury management of arthritis

- Joint repair and reconstruction, including contracture release and management of stiff joints

- Management of congenital deformities, including syndactyly, polydactyly, radia aplasia, and others

- Management of fingertip injuries

- Management of fractures and dislocations, including phalangeal or metacarpal with and without internal fixation; carpus, radius, and ulna with and without internal fixation; and injuries to joints and ligaments

- Management of tumors of the bone and soft tissue

- Management of upper extremity vascular disorders and insufficiencies

- Nerve repair and reconstruction, including upper extremity peripheral nerves, nerve graft, neurolysis, neuroma management, nerve decompression, and transposition

- Osteonecrosis, including Kinebock's disease

- Replantation and revascularization

- Tendon sheath release

- Tendon transfer and tendon balancing

- Tenorrhaphy, including flexor tendon repair and graft, implantation of tendon spacer, extensor tendon repair, and tenolysis/tenodesis

- Thumb reconstruction, including pollicization, toe-hand transfer, and thumb metacarpal lengthening

- Treatment of thermal injuries

- Upper extremity pain management

- Wound closure, including skin grafts, tissue flaps (local, regional, and distant), and free microvascular tissue transfer

Burden on the Applicant

If a practitioner wishes to maintain clinical privileges, he or she must provide the medical staff services department with evidence that demonstrates current clinical competence. In short, he or she must ensure that the competence equation is answered to the department chair's and credentials committee's satisfaction. However, the practitioner in question may have difficulty providing this information if he or she has not recently provided care within the scope of privileges being requested. When a practitioner seeks clinical privileges but cannot provide evidence demonstrating his or her competence, it is not the medical staff services department's or credentials committee's responsibility to prove the practitioner is competent. It is the practitioner's responsibility to prove that he or she meets the minimum threshold criteria established by the medical staff for the clinical privileges he or she requested.

Department chairs should not hesitate to alert the credentials committee and MEC when they are unable to assess a physician's current clinical competence due to the absence of information. The department chair, credentials committee, or MEC must use its experience, skills, and knowledge to respond appropriately. In such situations, the organization typically has already assessed whether the practitioner meets established criteria for membership and/or clinical privileges, but the applicant or department chair may need to modify the physician's request for clinical privileges. In any case, the organization should place the burden on the applicant to provide information that resolves all doubt about his or her competence to perform the requested privileges. For the purposes of this chapter, the tip below is applicable in selective practice scenarios related to the physician who has narrowed his or her practice.

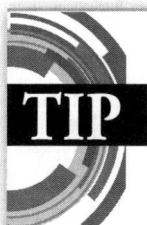

TIP

Credentials committees often overanalyze credentialing and privileging decisions regarding low- and no-volume practitioners in an attempt to avoid insulting or criticizing a colleague. However, the best course of action is to approach every applicant in a businesslike manner. Rely on your policies and procedures to avoid the appearance of impropriety, and communicate with the low- or no-volume practitioner regarding:

- Established criteria for clinical privileges, including whether your facility requires a minimum number of patient contacts per year

- The physician's plans to grow or narrow his or her practice

- The hospital's increased focus on determining proficiency for clinical privileges

- Your medical staff's strategic direction

- Volumes incurred at your facility

Revisiting Specialized Medical Center

Going back to our case study, the medical staff leaders and administration at Specialized Medical Center recognize that there is no single solution to address the issue of selective practice affecting physicians' ability to maintain competence for the full set of core privileges and, therefore, ED call coverage. They identify the following statements as their foundation for addressing this issue:

1. Credentialing has no master other than the patient. Any decisions related to credentialing and privileging, whether it be policy development or recommendations and actions taken on requests for clinical privileges, will be made in the best interest of patient safety.

2. A commitment to hospital success and physician success. To provide quality patient care and meet both community and physician needs, efforts to solve the issue of selective practice must focus on the success of the hospital and of the physician.

3. Specialized Medical Center has specific obligations to meet EMTALA requirements.

They then decide on the following action items to assist in managing those goals:

- Educate all medical staff leaders on EMTALA requirements.

- Recognize that all practitioners are permitted privileges in an emergency situation to protect life and limb of the patient, as outlined in medical staff governance documents (bylaws, policies and procedures, rules and regulations, privilege forms, etc.).

- Evaluate current ED call obligations and determine which practitioners are required to serve call

- Address ED call obligations and privileges separately by establishing an MEC policy for ED call by specialty and accurately defining clinical privileges and linking those privileges to current competency before granting privileges to a practitioner.

- Accurately delineate clinical privileges through creating privileging "clusters" as applicable.

- Add the following sample language to privilege forms or include it in an MEC call policy: Assess, stabilize, and determine the disposition of patients with emergent conditions consistent

 The Medical Staff's Guide to Overcoming Competence Assessment Challenges

with medical staff policy regarding emergency and consultative call services. (If your organization uses a core privileging system, include the statement within the core description of the specialty.)

- Continually reassess whether practitioners can meet this minimum expectation or need to provide alternative coverage.